THE BELLY MAPPING® METHOD

A gentle, creative guide to feel baby's position and bond in pregnancy

From the creator of Spinning Babies®
Gail Tully, Midwife
Minnesota, USA

The Belly Mapping® Method: A gentle, creative guide to feel baby's position and bond in pregnancy
Gail N. Tully
1959-
Includes Bibliographical references and glossodex.

Electronic PDF
ISBN: 978-0-9908307-7-1

Print Edition
ISBN: 978-1-7357489-1-7
  1. family
  2. health

Library of Congress Control Number: 2025917803

Previously published as The Belly Mapping® Workbook; How kicks and wiggles reveal baby's position.
Copyright © 2005, 2006, 2010, by Maternity House Publishing, Inc., the parent company of Spinning Babies®.

Special thanks to Ruthie Nelson for editing and Megan Stark for designing the book layout and cover.

Credits: Front and back cover photos by Kristen Tangen, www.facebook.com/kristintangenphotography
All illustrations and photographs inside the book are by Gail Tully and the following contributors, alphabetical by last name:
Banerjee family, p. 68 (bottom).
Candace Barber, pp. 1; 7; 8; 14 (small photo); 17; 30; 31 (top left); 41 (top right).
Jenny Blyth, pp. 88 (left); 91.
Czarina Bowers, pp. 5; 11; 99; 101.
Sue Damgaard, pp. 107 (top); 108 (top).
Todd Ernst, p.67.
Jessica Freeman, p. 106.
Trish Gardiner, pp. 65; 102 (right); 104 (bottom); 114.
Brian Garland, pp. 6; 34 (top).
Jackie Goulart Fotographia, pp. 55; 69; 85.
Robin Martin, p. 86 (the three studio pictures).
Chris McBride, pp. 17 (top two right); 32 (top); 41 (top left and bottom); 50, 53: 54; 59; 82 top left; 83; 105 (top); 108 (bottom); 109; 111 (top).
Sylvia Muda, p. 88 (center).
Philip Perkhov, p. 111 (bottom).
LaToshia Rouse, p. 103; 106.
Patience Salgado, p. 38 (top right)
Megan Stark, p. 38 (Bobo).
Kristen Tangen, pp. 14; 15; 29; 32 (bottom); 37; 38 (top); 45; 62 (top); 82 (bottom left); 87 (bottom); 88 (right); 92; 93; 97; 100; 102 (left).
Jennifer Walker, pp. 62 (bottom); 105 (bottom); 107 (bottom).
Catherine Warren, In the Moment Photography, pp. 13; 41 (middle right); 42; 43; 98.
Valerie Wiesner, p. 94.
Unknown Name, p. 34 (middle), 66 (parent email), 68 (top); 82 - pic of Gail painting at a Spinning Babies® event.
Stock photos are on pp. 4; 19; 92; 93.
AI: enhancement of Gail's photo on p. 87;

Every effort has been made to obtain proper permission to use the images. In the event that any acknowledgment has been inadvertently omitted, all necessary corrections will be made in future printings.

All rights reserved. No part of this book may be reproduced or transmitted in any form or by any means, electrical or mechanical, including photocopying or recording or by any information storage and retrieval system, without the written permission of the author, except for the inclusion of brief quotations in a review.

These descriptions for determining fetal position may not be entirely successful for every pregnant woman. How an individual applies these techniques may be more or less precise; the mother may have unique attributes to her anatomy, and/ or the fetus can change positions. Birth outcomes cannot be guaranteed for any individual, and descriptions are general and fit groups, not individuals. Parents and caregivers are encouraged to support a physiologically spontaneous labor and birth when possible and safe, and to decide together what, and when, interventions may be needed. Although the author and publisher have made every effort to ensure that the information in this book is accurate and current, only your caregiver knows you only your caregiver knows you and your health history well enough to make specific recommendations. The authors, editors, reviewers, and publisher disclaim any liability from use of this book.

The descriptions for determining fetal position may not be entirely successful for every pregnant woman. How an individual applies these techniques may be more or less precise, the mother may have unique attributes to her anatomy, and/or the fetus can change positions. Birth outcomes cannot be guaranteed for any individual, and descriptions are general and fit groups, not individuals. Parents and caregivers are encouraged to support a physiologically spontaneous labor and birth when possible and safe, and to decide together what, and when, interventions may be needed. Although the author and publisher have made every effort to ensure that the information in this book is accurate and current, only your caregiver knows you and your health history well enough to make specific recommendations. The author, editors, reviewers, and publisher disclaim any liability from use of this book.

PRAISE FOR
THE BELLY MAPPING® METHOD

"The Belly Mapping® Method is a beautiful way to bridge the gap between medical care and emotional connection.
By encouraging parents to get curious, to listen,
and to creatively engage with their baby in the womb, we honor both the science and the spirit of pregnancy. This integrated approach nurtures the whole family, before and beyond birth.
-Phyllis Klaus, PsyD, DONA Founder

"...an incredibly valuable piece of work ... highly interesting for expectant parents as well as for healthcare providers involved in prenatal care."
-Sylvia Muda, SpB®CPE, Fysiotherapiemuda.nl

"Gail Tully combines unique gifts of clinical expertise, experience, creativity, sensitivity, intuition, original thinking, and wisdom to solve the mysteries of the baby's position in utero. She shows pregnant women and their caregivers a variety of clues that reveal the baby position and
how to put them all together to create a picture of the baby inside."
- Penny Simkin, PT, DONA Founder

"What a gem of a book! The Belly Mapping® Method is a delightful invitation to get to know your baby before birth. What I love most is how it turns curiosity and gentle touch into real bonding—building trust, joy, and connection while your baby is still inside. This method offers a simple, sweet way to feel more confident and more in love as you prepare to meet your tiniest New One."
-Carrie Contey, PhD author of CALMS: A Guide to Soothing Your Baby

"I wish every person expecting a baby could enjoy Gail Tully's Belly Mapping® Method book. Her book is extraordinary, and I found it fun.
My granddaughter is soon to be married, when she embarks upon the journey into motherhood, I'll be giving her a copy of this wonderful book.
May all pregnancies and births be blessed.
-Ibu Robin Lim, Midwife, grandmother, activist for reproductive justice and Peace on Earth

Belly Mapping® Method invites parents into a deep connection with their unborn baby. This book reaffirms that parents and babies are active participants together in their experience of pregnancy and birth—an important cornerstone of prenatal and perinatal psychology.
-Association for Prenatal and Perinatal Psychology and Health (APPPAH)

"...A wonderfully intimate way for a mother to help connect with her baby in the womb as well as have a sense of baby's position. The information in this slim volume will make a world of difference in your comfort for pregnancy and birth."
-Robin Elise Weiss, BA, CLC, ICCE-CPE, CD(DONA), LCCE, FACCE, and About.com Guide to Pregnancy/Birth

Here's What You'll Learn in this Book

Before You Begin
- How to Use This Book.. 2
- An Overview of the 3 Steps... 3
- How Your Provider Finds Your Baby by Feel... 7
- Know Your Parts, Know Your Baby's Parts... 8, 9

Prenatal Bonding.. 10, 36, 44, 52, 64, 84, 96

Step 1: Map Your Belly
Feeling and writing down where you feel your baby's head, trunk, and limbs............ 11
- What Are the Marks on the Map?... 12
- Feeling Your Belly... 13
- Which Direction is Baby Lying? Vertical Lie, Transverse Lie, Oblique Lie...... 15
- Are Those Little Parts the Hands Fluttering or the Feet Kicking?......... 18
- Finding Baby's Head.. 21
- Before You Draw a Map, Give Easy Answers... 23
- Your Turn... 25
- Sensation Maps for the Belly Mapping® Method................................... 26
- Frequently Asked Questions.. 31
- Anterior Placenta.. 32
- Tracking Baby's Position Changes... 33

Step 2: Visualize Your Baby
Put a doll over your belly, or have a belly painting, to "see" your baby's position........ 37
- Parents Using a Doll to Visualize Baby's Position................................... 41
- The Night The Belly Mapping® Method Was Proven............................. 42

Step 3: Name Baby's Position
Learn your baby's position name to understand the terms and prepare for labor...... 45
- Name Baby's Position.. 46
- Fetal Position Names and You... 50
- What Is Your Baby's Position?.. 51

The Belly Mapping® Method for a Breech Baby
Tips and details; photos of a pregnant mother discovering the baby's head is up..... 53

The Belly Mapping® Method With Twins
Twice as tricky, but twice the fun... 65

How Baby's Position Affects Your Labor
Explore how different baby positions might influence labor....................... 69

What to Do and Who Can Help
Get a proactive approach to support baby's position and your labor progress..... 85

Games to Play with Your Baby... 91

Belly Painting: Bonus Section.. 97

Appendix... 109

Glossodex... 115

Welcome!

Welcome to The Belly Mapping® Method. You are about to begin a compassionate and empowering experience.

Who is the little guest growing inside you?

Since 2004, I've guided parents in seeing their babies by touch through the creation of The Belly Mapping® Method.

Why? Because parents and doulas asked, "Why didn't my birth team know my baby's position?"

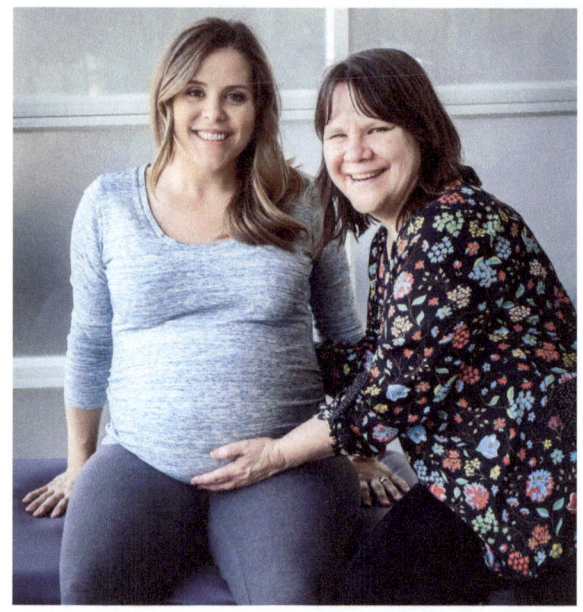

The Belly Mapping® Method puts the know-how into your own hands—literally.

Welcome to a new way of connecting to yourself, your body, and your baby.

♡ Gail

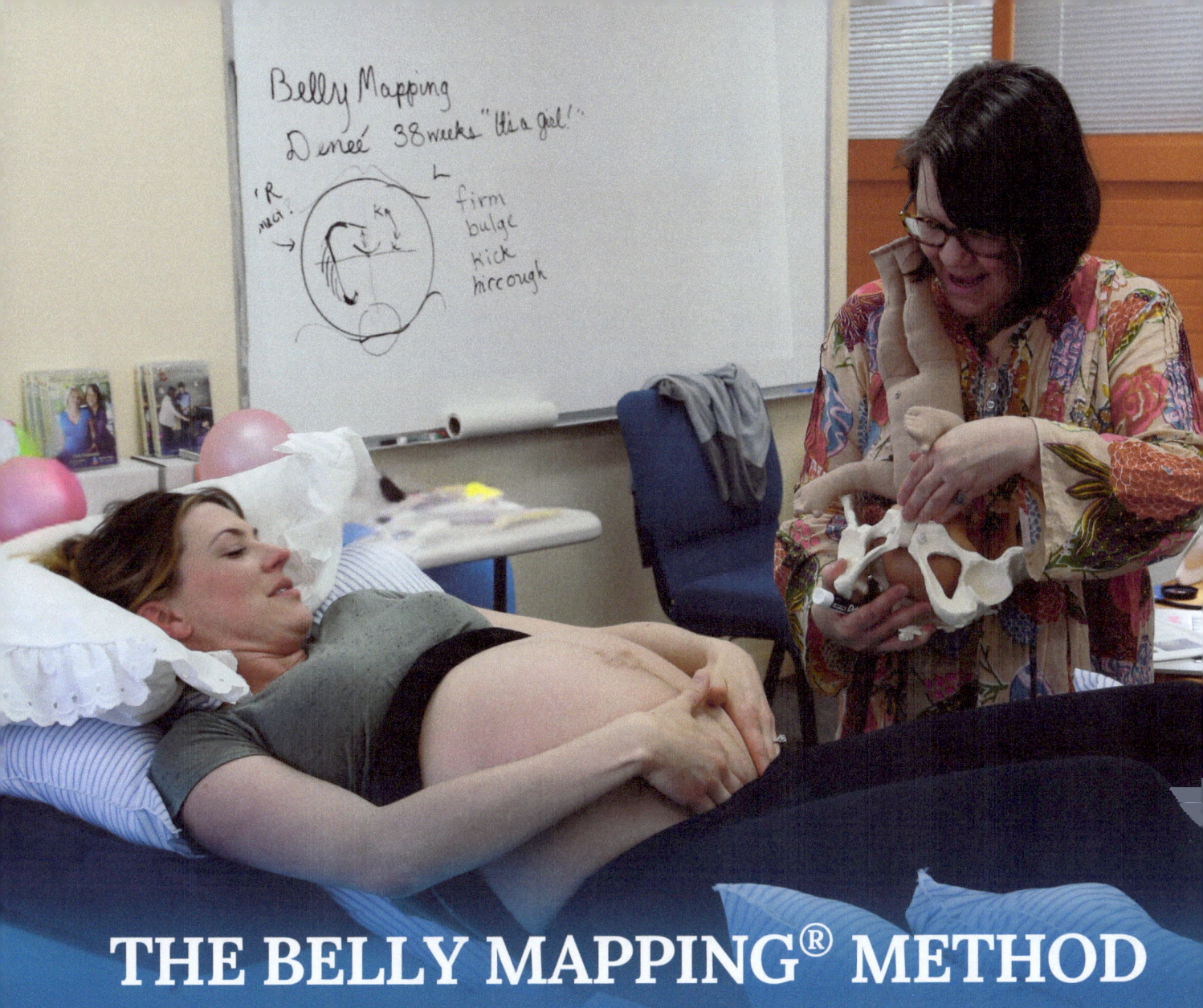

THE BELLY MAPPING® METHOD

Before You Begin

Please have fun with your learning. Don't worry about being accurate. Just enjoy feeling your baby at first. Begin with awareness. Your mind will catch up later.

Your baby enjoys your touch. Be curious about how your baby responds. Babies respond slowly. Breathing slowly will help you tune into your baby's pace.

Let yourself have a sense of humor. "Mother's laugh is baby's joy."

How to Use This Book

While reading this book, keep your eyes open for birth geek-speak in **_bold italics_**. You'll find all these words in the **Glossodex** at the end of the book.

 Where you see teacups, Gail shares her friendly insights, like she's sharing a cup of tea with you.

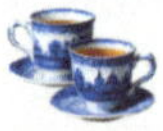

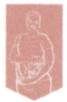 In the pink, Chris McBride, birth doula and administrative doula to world-renowned therapist Phyllis Klaus, shares highlights of prenatal bonding.

Many parents enjoy seeing their baby drawn on their belly after discovering the baby's position. A bonus painting guide is at the end of this book, which may help your friend paint your belly.

Record your discoveries in this book or **download** the free template maps found via the QR code to the right.

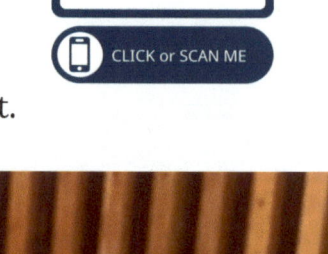

Read Step 1 through quickly first, then read it while you do it. You may like to bring this book along to a prenatal appointment.

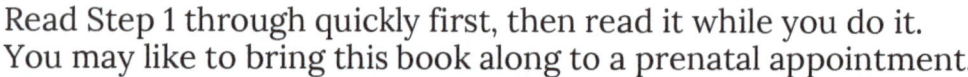

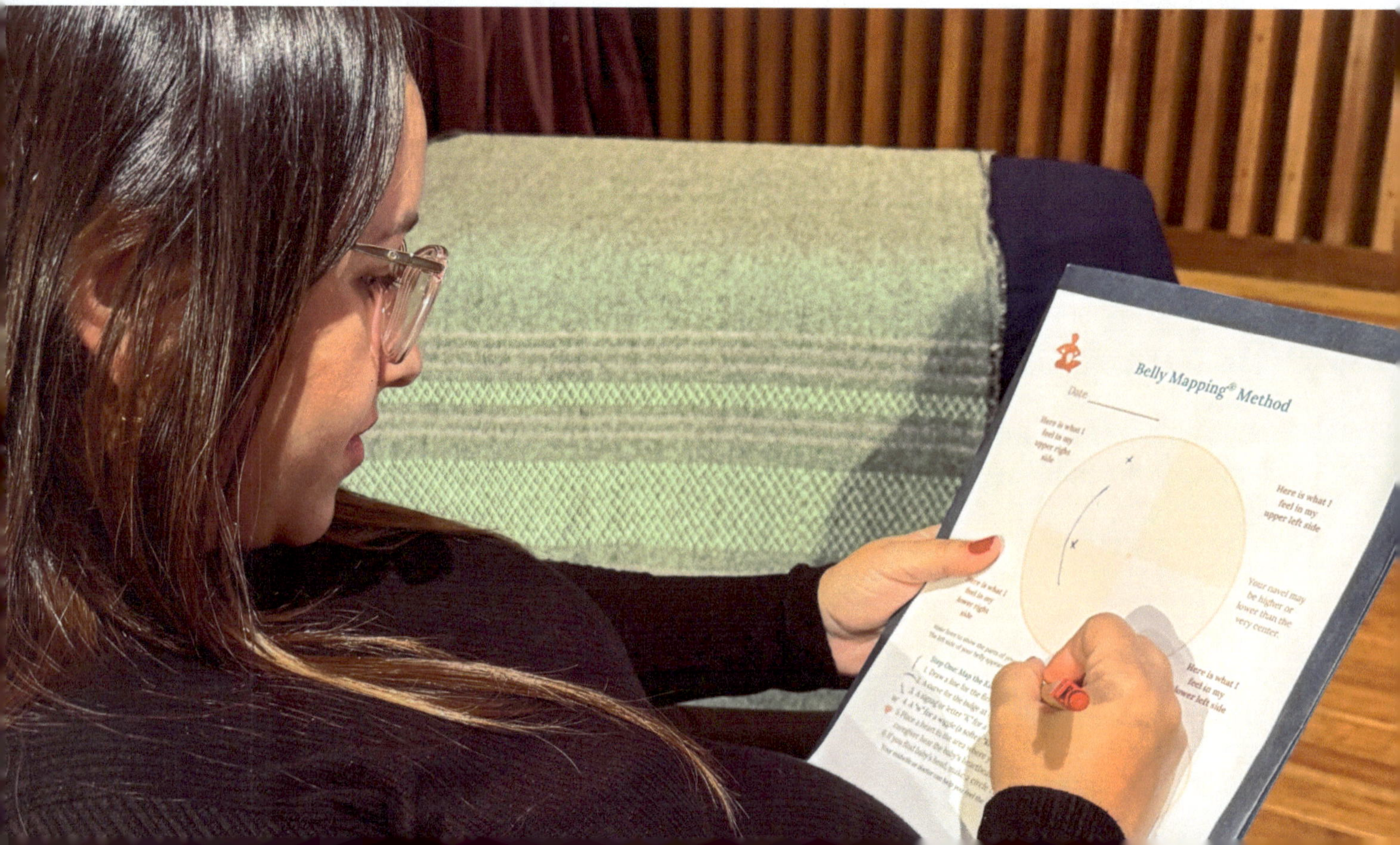

An Overview of the Three Steps

Consider the many details of figuring out your baby's position as three simple steps. Taking things step-by-step makes something potentially complex into a fun experience for you—and your baby. Baby gets a cuddle while you explore!

Step 1: Map Your Belly

Step 2: Visualize Your Baby

Step 3: Name Baby's Position

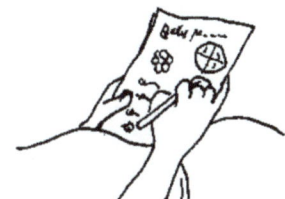

Going one step at a time is easier than everything all at once. When feeling your belly, you feel parts of your baby and yourself. That's a lot. Try one area at a time.

We draw the abdomen in quadrants as a simpler way to note where we find baby's parts. A fifth, round area at the bottom is just to see if hands are there.

In Step 1, you'll mark the areas where there's baby action.

In Step 2, you'll link them back together again to get a sense of how your baby's body is inside your womb.

Some readers are interested only in these first two steps.

Step 3 can reveal the fetal position name. Empower your name knowledge to use our materials for guiding you through labor and to speak "birth talk" with your midwife or doctor.

No one will have to ask, "Why didn't anybody know!?"

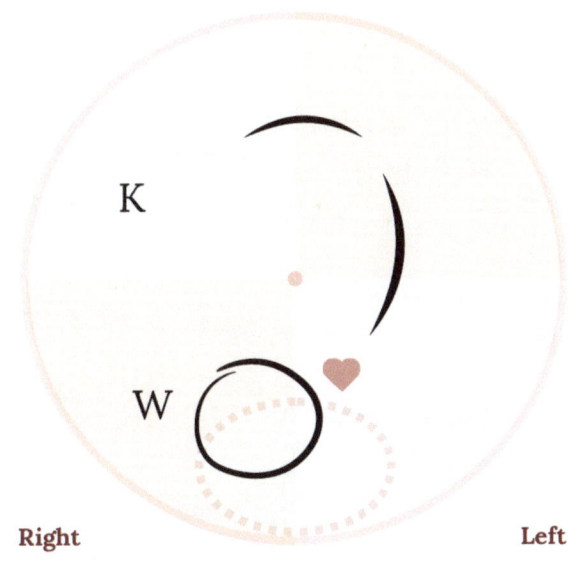

The map of baby's position you create in Step 1 shows how to hold the doll in Step 2 and guides you in naming the position in Step 3.

You can find clues for filling out your map described in the Step 1 chapter. Read "How Baby's Position Affects Labor" on page 69.

The Belly Mapping® Method: A Path to Prenatal Bonding

Prenatal bonding is the emotional connection you have with your gestating baby.

Bonding is a term from the famous pediatrician partners Marshall Klaus and John Kennell for the emotional connection of a parent with their child.

Research in prenatal and **perinatal** psychology shows that our womb experiences impact our entire lives.

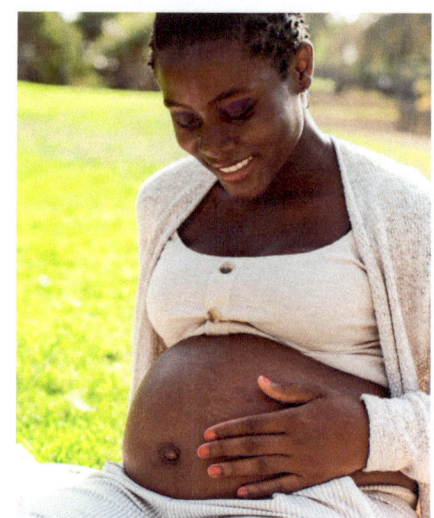

How well do you already know your baby in this pregnancy? Some parents expect their child to have specific characteristics, while others may feel like a tiny stranger is entering their lives. This process invites exploration of your actual, real baby: a person with their own being. A more secure attachment is the reward!

Attune to your parenting with open joy during your child's most vulnerable stage of development. New creative abilities strengthen this secure bond with your baby.

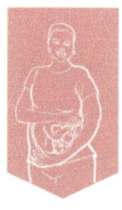

Look throughout the book for sections describing the benefits of bonding, which include:

1. Establishing Secure Connection
2. Embracing Creativity
3. Cultivating Confidence
4. Opening to Love
5. Communicating Kindness
6. Awakening Inner Wisdom
7. Inviting Bliss

Including a Partner

The Belly Mapping® Method can be between you and your baby, or you can invite special people to be with you. The Belly Mapping® Method is a way to help loved ones understand and celebrate the unique human being growing inside!

Often, the first thing a partner wants to know is whether touching the baby is safe. Gently following these instructions with a soft touch is safe. Using the pads of the fingers to slowly press onto baby ensures baby's comfort and safety.

"...Belly Mapping was such a wonderful opportunity to connect to each other and imagine together what it will be like to meet our sweet beanie bundle! This was both informative and exciting, and we would highly recommend doing a Belly Mapping session for any expecting couple."

–Cassandra and Daniel Dagones

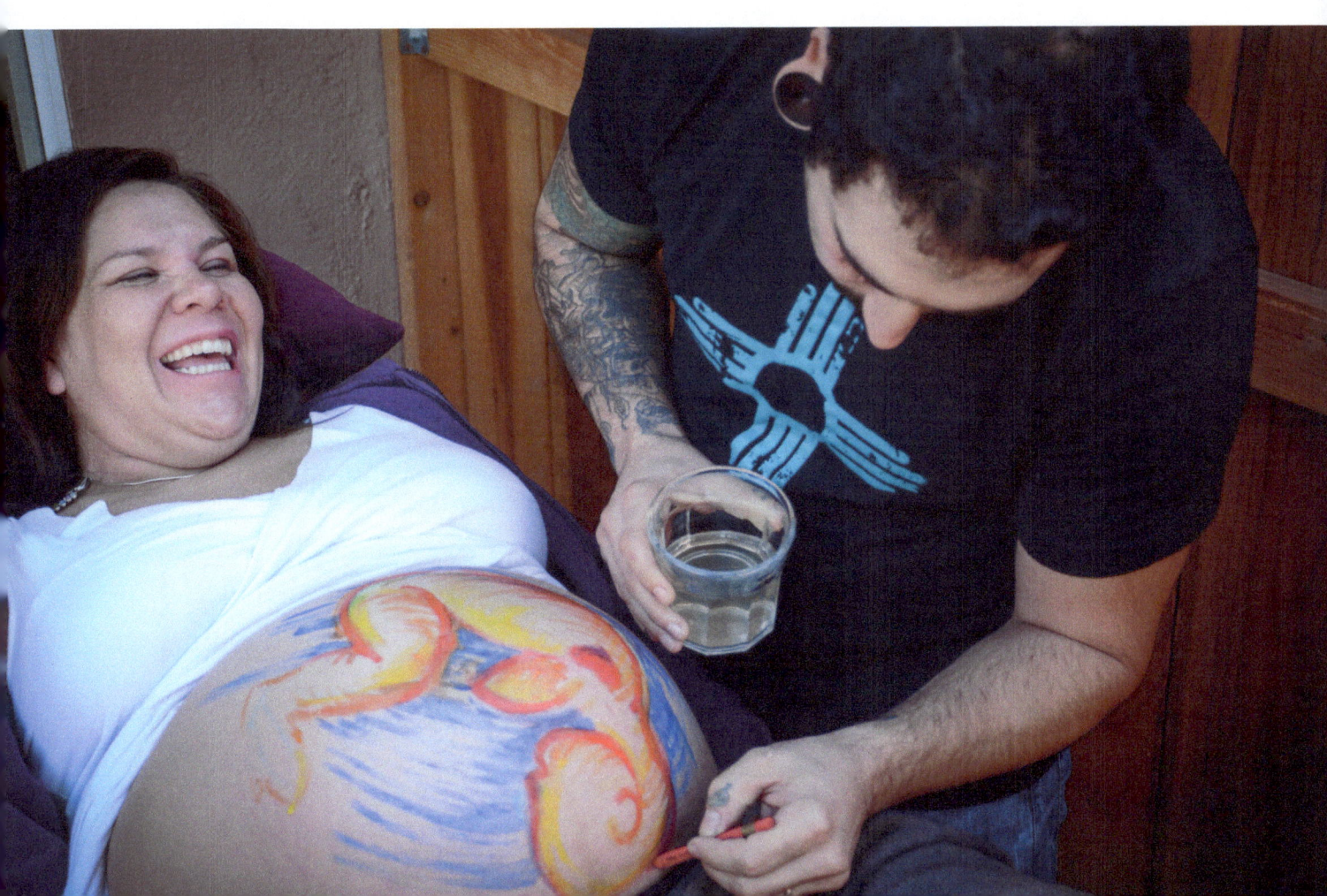

When to Start

The Belly Mapping® Method is easier in the last trimester, sometime after 28 weeks.

The further along you are, the easier it is to feel your baby as the abdomen softens.

Earlier in pregnancy, you may be able to tell which direction your baby is lying in the womb. You might be able to notice a few more details late in the second trimester. If you are eager to start before the third trimester, you may still discover some fun details.

Try The Belly Mapping® Method just before you drift to sleep. This is a time when your pregnant belly relaxes and lets you feel your baby's wiggles and kicks.

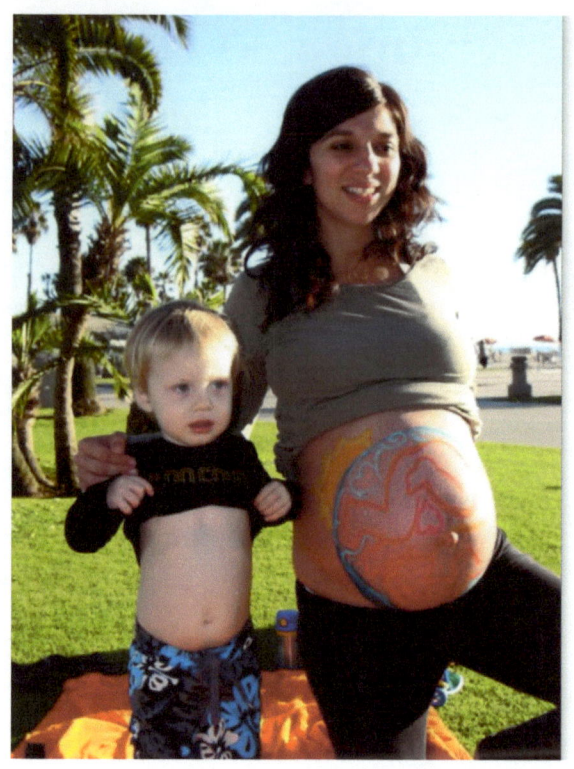

Get Comfortable!
Lie down to feel your baby. Lying down lets your abdomen drape softly over your baby. Bend your legs and put a pillow under your knees to relax your belly even more while increasing your comfort.

Prop yourself up a little. You can tilt your back slightly to the side if you feel odd while on your back. Place a pillow under your right shoulder and hip to tilt to the left side. (Typically, the left side is best, but choose the side you're more comfortable on.) If you feel uncomfortable, change position or try again later.

How easy it is to feel your baby, and how accurate, depends on your position, muscle tone, body fat, and amount of amniotic fluid. Standing or sitting makes your tummy too tight to feel details. Lie down! You can't feel your baby if you lift your head to look!

When you're ready, a template can be downloaded and printed for **Step 1: Map Your Baby**.

How Your Care Provider Finds Your Baby by Feel

Doctors, nurses, and midwives are taught to feel (**palpate**) the pregnant abdomen in four hand positions, called **Leopold's Maneuvers**. They might find parts of the baby and amniotic fluid, and, once in a while, they'll feel the spongy, thick **placenta**. Palpating is what a midwife, doctor, or nurse does. It is care provider centered. The Belly Mapping® Method is what pregnant parents do, and it is parent centered.

These hand positions help answer four helpful questions:
1. What is at the top of the uterus?
2. What is on the sides?
3. What part of the baby is **presenting** at the top opening of the pelvis?
4. Is the presenting part **engaged**? If it is a head, is the head **flexed** or **extended**?

 Assumptions may lead to mistaking a hip for a head during Question 3. Many **care providers** simply skip Question 4.

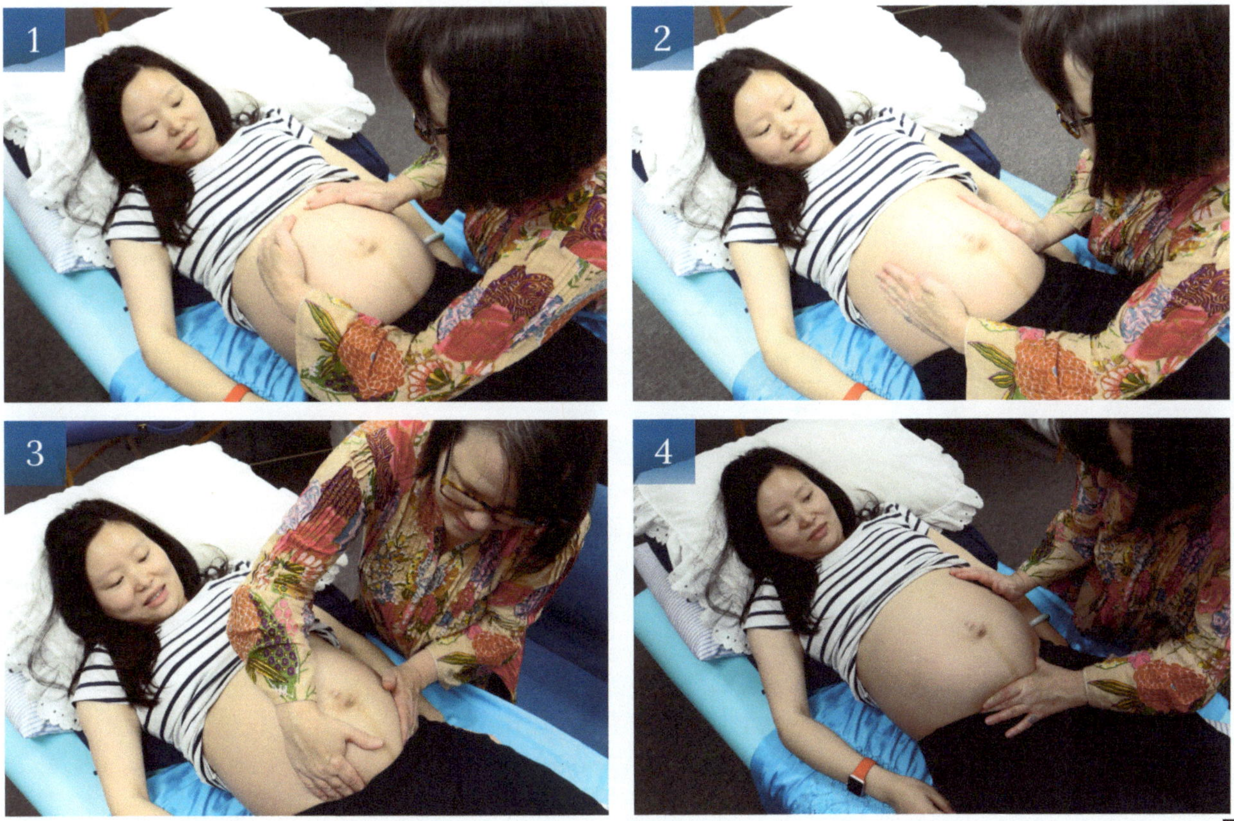

Know Your Parts

Feeling your body parts also helps you know which parts are you and which parts are the baby. While this might seem obvious, it's not! The parts of you that are useful for The Belly Mapping® Method include:

- The top of the uterus, or **fundus**.
- The very front of the pelvis, often called the **pubic bone** (symphysis pubis).
- Your navel!
- The **linea nigra** is a vertical line that develops in pregnancy as a temporary pigmented stripe from the navel to the pubic bone. This "center line" divides the right and left of your abdomen.

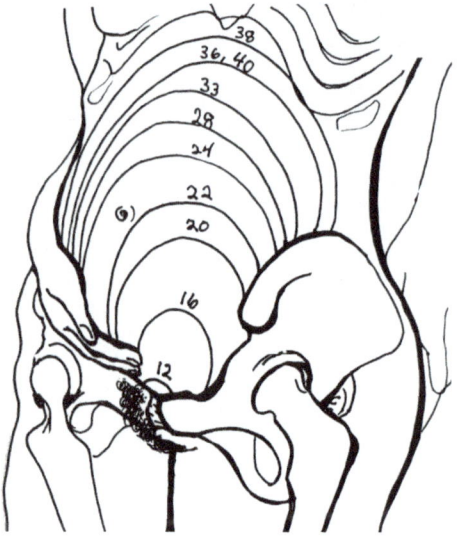

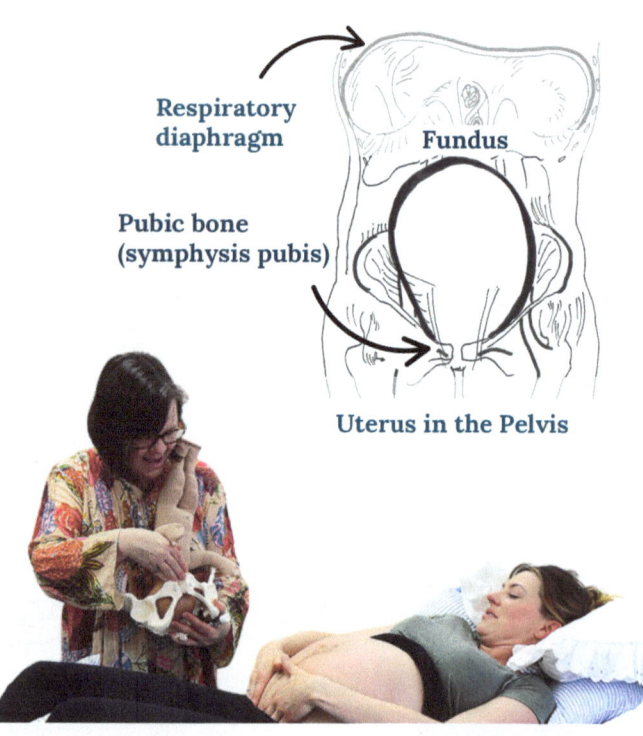

Uterine Size at Weeks of Pregnancy
This sketch shows the general idea for you.

- The top of the uterus comes to the top of the pubic bone (but deeper) at 12 weeks gestation.
- The uterus is level with the navel at about 20–22 weeks pregnant.
- By 36 weeks, the navel is at the center of your map.
- The uterus drops when baby engages (38 weeks or in labor).

Note the angle is ¾ view, not frontal.

Gather Clues from Your Prenatal Appointment
Your midwife or doctor will note baby's head position during the exam, whether they feel by hand or by **ultrasound**. Ask for help to feel baby's head and bum.

The heartbeat may be heard lower than your navel when baby is **head down** and above your navel for a **breech**. A Doppler ultrasound detects the heartbeat from far away, whereas a **fetoscope** (fetal stethoscope) has to be on baby's back to pick up the beat. Draw a heart where the heartbeat is found to remember.

8

Know Baby's Parts

Looking at a baby, their parts are quite obvious: a head, a body, arms, legs, hands, and feet. Why would we need to review such common knowledge?

Because when baby is hidden under your abdomen, their parts suddenly seem mysterious!

You'll notice baby's kicks tapping against the inside of your abdomen. Baby's back is the longest, smoothest part. Baby is all curled up, cute as a button!

Baby's head may be tucked out of reach, deep in your pelvis. Or it may be up by your heart.

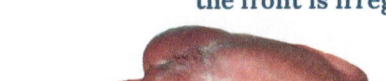

The back is smooth; the front is irregular.

Two feet together make a bulge!

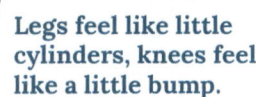

Legs feel like little cylinders, knees feel like a little bump.

You'll notice there are no cylinders (thighs) coming from the head.

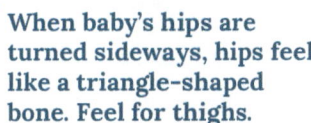

When baby's hips are turned sideways, hips feel like a triangle-shaped bone. Feel for thighs.

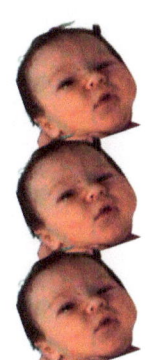

36+ cm flexed

35 cm flexed

A baby's body is twice the length of baby's head.

The head and hips of a full-term baby are close to the same width. Hips turned toward the front can feel like a head.

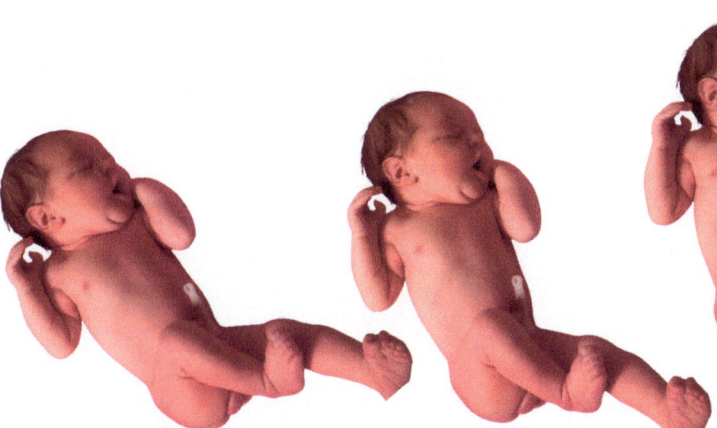

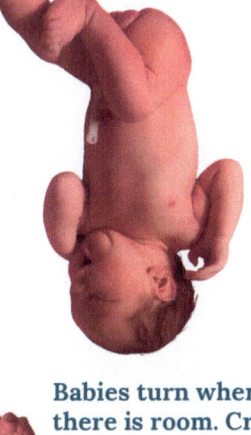

Babies turn when there is room. Create room with balance.

Baby's hands often move by the mouth or ears. An arm moves differently than a leg.

Baby's feet kick out and pull back in.

Baby's knees can come up by their tummies.

Establishing Secure Connection
The Power of Prenatal Bonding to Overcome Fear

A comprehensive study of 255 first-time mothers found that as prenatal bonding increased, fear of childbirth significantly decreased.[1] Women who felt more connected to their babies during pregnancy reported less anxiety and greater confidence about labor and delivery.[1,2,3]

This emotional connection reshapes the experience of birth, fostering trust in your body and transforming fear into anticipation. Viewing birth as a shared journey with your baby helps you approach labor with greater calm and assurance.

Three Practices to Establish a Secure Connection
One beautiful thing about prenatal bonding is that during pregnancy, you can strengthen your relationship with your baby at any moment:

1. **Write** a letter to your baby, starting with the sentiment, *Welcome home*. Tell them all about the ways you are preparing to meet them.
2. **Imagine** the umbilical cord delivering love and comfort along with nutrition. Place your hands on your belly; breathe deeply. Use your imagination to visualize your connection to your baby flowing with a deep feeling of security.
3. **Breathe** in deeply. Inhale and imagine joy, happiness, and calm filling your whole body. Each breath gives your baby good oxygen. Exhale slowly, empty your lungs completely, and consciously push out all remaining air.

Your Journey Forward
As you continue through your pregnancy, remember that every moment you spend connecting with your baby is an investment in well-being for both of you.

During moments of quiet meditation, rest your hands on your belly. Feel the love and confidence, building a foundation that will serve you in birth and beyond.

Your body and your baby's body are designed for this incredible journey.

By nurturing your connection now, you're beginning the beautiful adventure of parenthood with the deep knowing that you and your baby are in this together.

References
1. Gürsoy, B., & Palas Karaca, P. (2025). The relationship between fear of birth and prenatal attachment and childbirth self-efficacy perception in primigravida women. *BMC Pregnancy and Childbirth*, 25(1), 462. https://doi.org/10.1186/s12884-025-07555-7
2. Smorti, M., Ponti, L., Simoncini, T., Pancetti, F., Mauri, G., & Gemignani, A. (2020). Psychological factors and maternal-fetal attachment in relation to epidural choice. *Midwifery*, 88, 102762. https://doi.org/10.1016/j.midw.2020.102762
3. Yin, A., Shi, Y., Heinonen, S., Räisänen, S., Fang, W., Jiang, H., & Chen, A. (2024). The impact of fear of childbirth on mode of delivery, postpartum mental health and breastfeeding: A prospective cohort study in Shanghai, China. *Journal of Affective Disorders*, 347, 183–191. https://doi.org/10.1016/j.jad.2023.11.054

Step #1
Map Your Baby

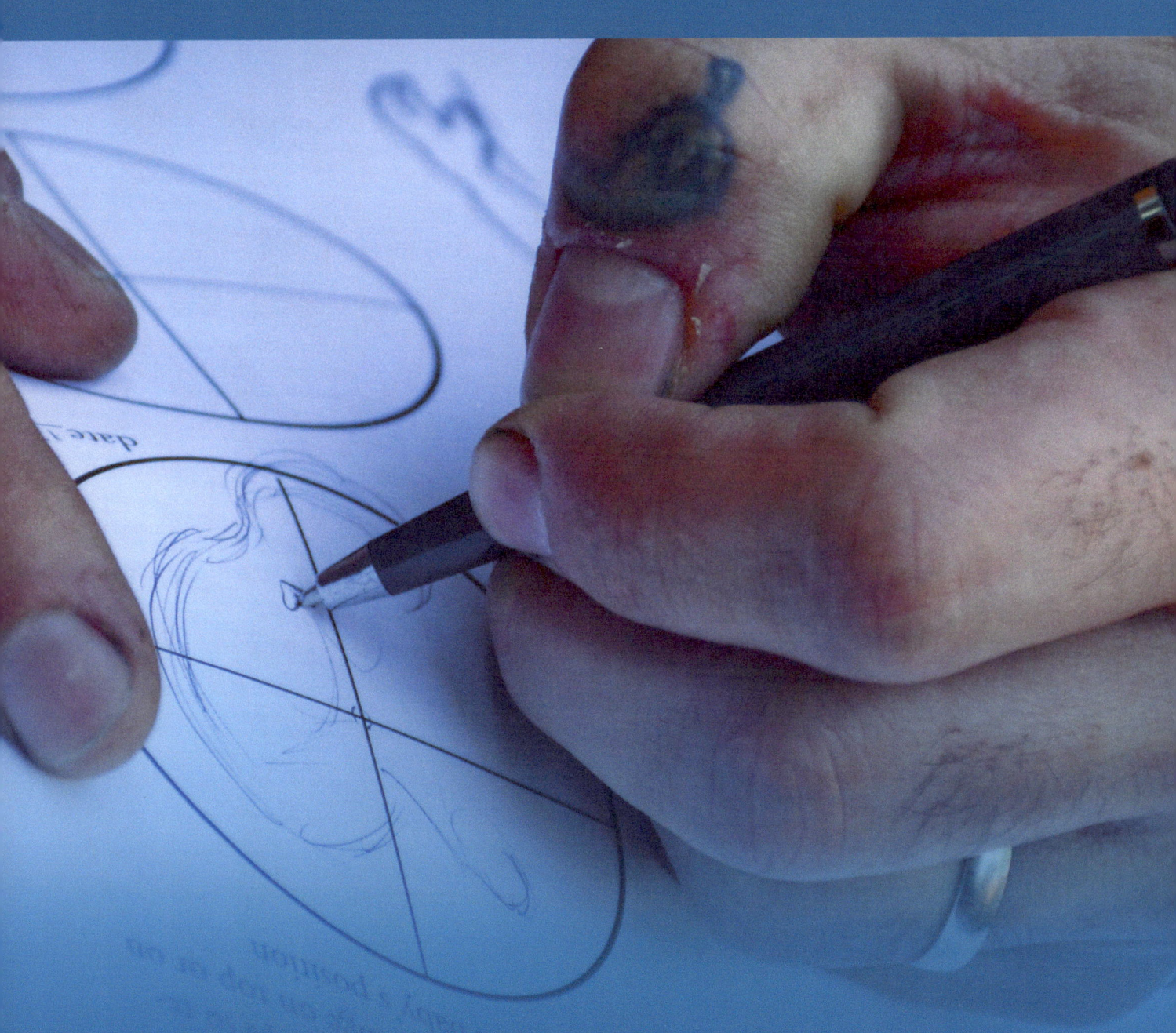

What Are the Marks on the Map?

At first, you'll just feel the little bumps that rise up when baby kicks and the larger, firm parts of their body. This page shows you how we map your baby.

Take a minute to check out the circles below to help your brain go from "uh-oh" to an "aha" discovery.

- Two lines divide the belly into four areas, making it easier to tell the location of baby's movements.
- The horizontal line is the "navel line."
- The vertical line is the center line or linea nigra.
- Gray areas are solid parts of the baby.
- Small gray circles are smaller parts of the baby.
- Big gray spots are larger parts of the baby.
- Some firm parts cross over into two or more quadrants of your belly.

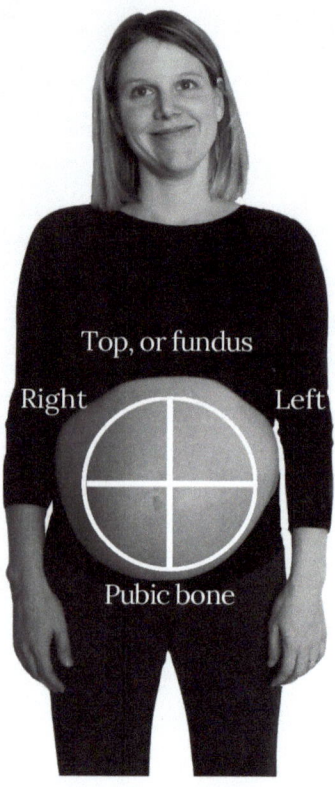

Mapping all the sensations may get overwhelming, so let's simplify it!

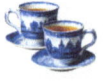 Maps are a mirror image of your belly. Your left side is on the right side of the paper, or map. Your right side is on the left side of the map.

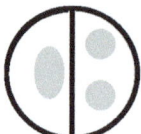

Big on the Right

Big parts are on the right, and small parts are on the left side of the belly.

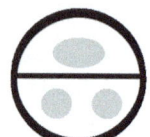

Biggest Above

More common earlier in pregnancy, the big part is over the small parts.

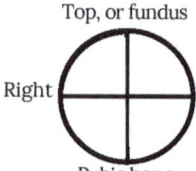

Less Detailed

Let's focus on four main areas of the abdomen. That's easier to map.

Take a Breath

You don't have to get this all at once. We will take you through The Belly Mapping® Method step-by-step. Follow these pages, and you are very likely to create a fairly accurate map of your baby's position. Skim through each chapter and then come back and read it as you go. You'll soon know baby's position!

Give yourself several tries. Keep it lighthearted; playing with baby is fun!

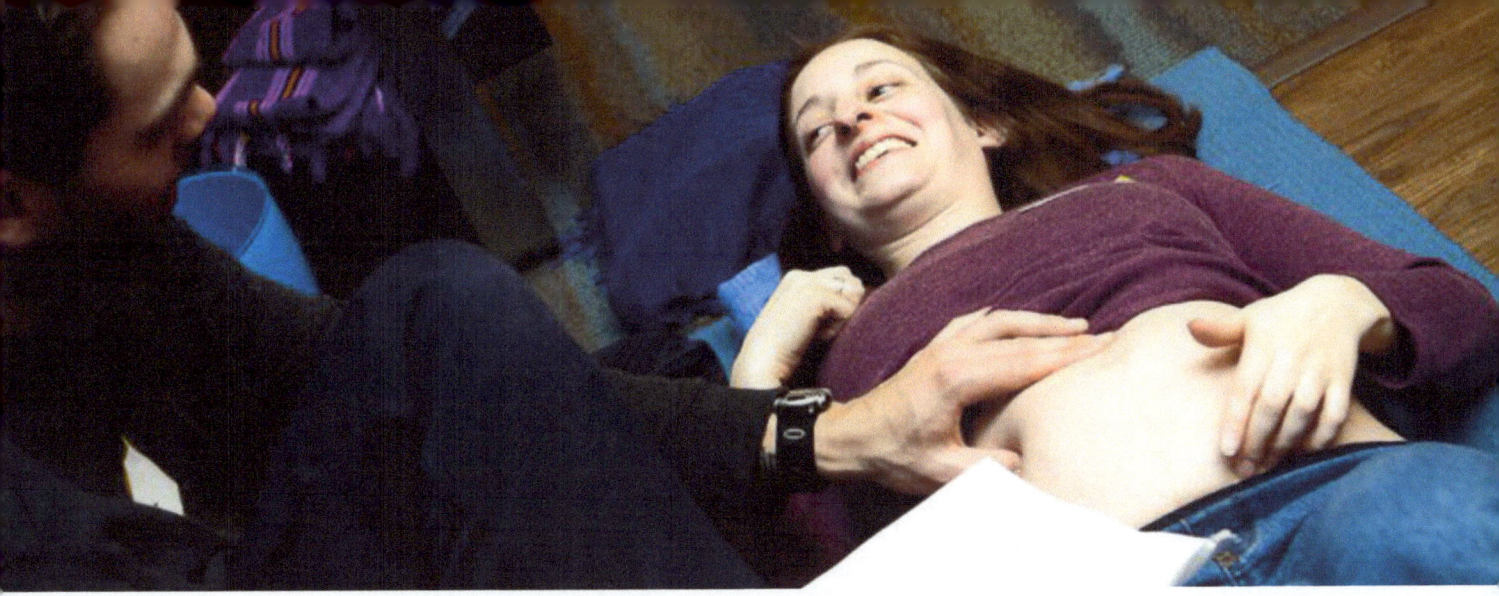

Step 1: Map Your Belly

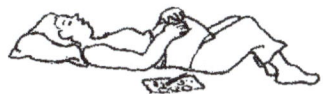

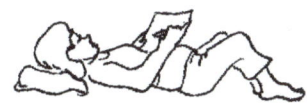

To make this easy, begin by reading all of Step 1. Then take your time to feel your baby's movements. Finally, read Step 1 again while you mark your map.

First, lie down so your abdomen relaxes over your baby. You can lie flat, or you can recline at a low angle. You may also tilt your back a little toward your left side so your uterus doesn't lay directly on your aorta.

Feeling Your Belly

Breathe deeply and sigh to soften your abdominal muscles. Wait for a contraction to end if your whole belly is hard. Then it will soften, allowing you to begin.

Once you're relaxed, press the pads of your fingers into your abdomen here and there until you find firmness. Feel a firm part that isn't you? Say hello to your baby!

Why **finger pads**? The fingerprint area of your fingers is highly sensitive and can be used to caress your baby, whereas poking with the fingertips doesn't give you the same sensitivity.

Here's a tip to "see" with your fingers: Pretend you have ink on your fingertips and you are making a print. You'll roll your fingers side to side. Making this same move while feeling your baby helps your fingers sense their shape.

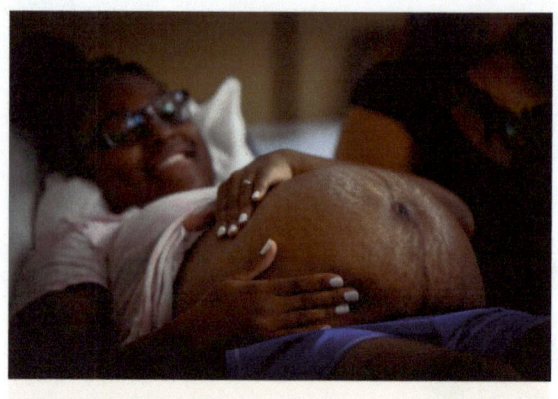
Is the Right Side Firm?

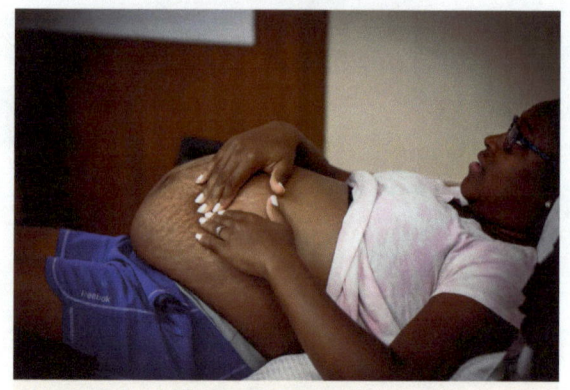
Is the Left Side Firm?

Think of Your Belly as Two Sides Inside a Circle
For now, just draw a circle on a sheet of paper. The circle represents the uterus. Later, use the template on page 25. That's your map.

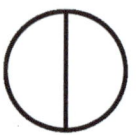

- Draw a vertical line in the middle of your circle. This line will be called the center line.

Which Side Is Firm? Which Side Is Soft?
You'll notice the round top (fundus) of your uterus is firmer than your belly just above it. The uterus has its own softer and firmer areas. Within the uterus, one area is firm where the baby is, while the other areas are soft with amniotic fluid.

After 32 weeks, one side of your belly may be noticeably firmer than the other. The firmness you feel is most likely the baby. Babies are rarely exactly in the middle.

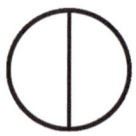 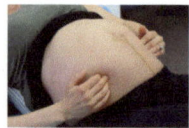

Soft and Firm

The uterus feels softer than the baby when there is no contraction.

 Baby, Water, or Placenta?
We assume soft areas are where there is amniotic fluid and firm areas are your baby. If the placenta is along the front wall of the uterus, you may feel the thick, spongy placenta (anterior placenta). Ask your care provider about the location of your placenta. See more about an anterior placenta on page 32.

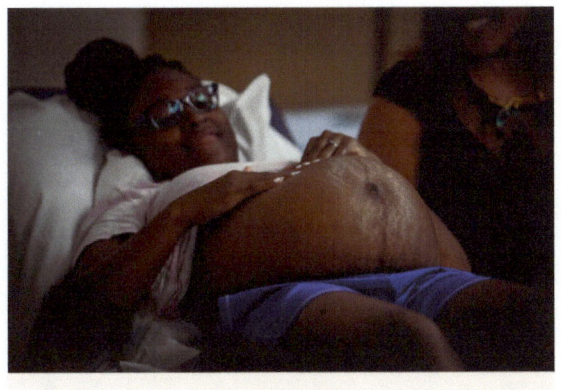
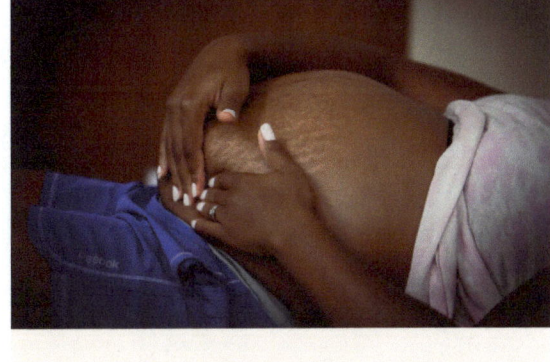

Top **Bottom**

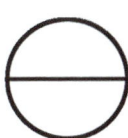

Top and Bottom
Now get to know how the top of your uterus feels in your abdomen.

Draw a horizontal line across the middle of your map. We will call this line the "navel line." Late in pregnancy, these lines cross at your navel.

Which Direction Is Baby Lying?
Once your fingers find the edges, or contours, of your baby's body, you'll notice the general direction in which the baby's body lies. The main body of the baby, or torso, is the largest firm part. On this page, you'll answer one question:

Is Baby Vertical, Sideways, or Diagonal?
You know your baby is vertical when the firmness of baby's body is longer from top to bottom in the uterus. There will be softness under your fingers along one or both sides of the baby's body. That's **amniotic fluid**. Head down is the most common position in the last half of pregnancy.

A **vertical lie** is when baby's spine matches the direction of your spine. We expect a baby to lie vertically just before the **third trimester** begins. Both head-down and head-up (breech) positions are in a vertical lie. A vertical baby can usually enter the pelvis.

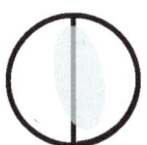

A **transverse lie** is when the baby is lying sideways in the womb. Their spine crosses from side to side, and the length of the baby stretches across the abdomen. Soft areas are above and below the baby at the top and bottom of your belly. Normal in early pregnancy but not later. Learn more on the next page.

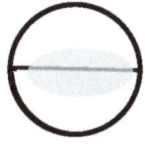

The **oblique lie** is when baby's head and body lie diagonally above the pelvis. Common in early pregnancy, not at the time of birth. Body balancing (page 62) often corrects a non-vertical lie.

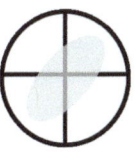

When Is a Transverse Lie Normal?
Baby's position is sideways in relation to the womb. This is normal in the first trimester. As the second trimester progresses, most babies will move into a vertical position, and most are head down by 26 weeks.

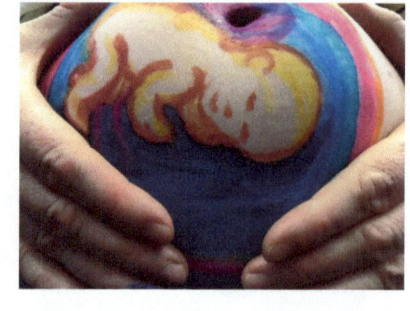

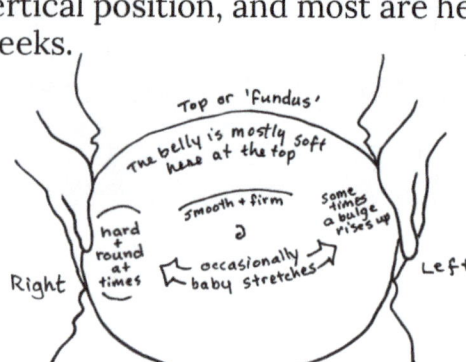

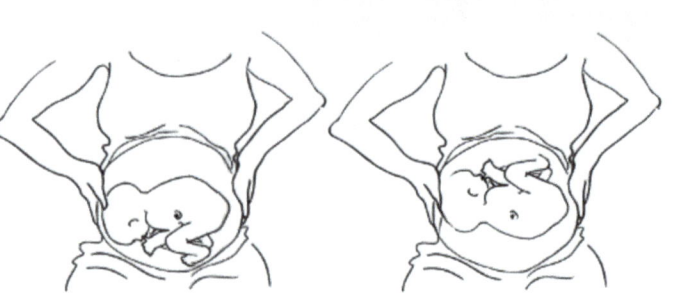

Uterine Torsion
The uterus can get a twist from a sudden jolt while turning, whether during sports, like swinging a bat or golf club, or a fall or car accident. **Uterine torsion** is not normal. Jensen (1992) noticed babies were often stuck in a transverse lie. A twist narrows the lower uterus, causing baby to lie sideways above it.

What Can Be Done?
Help baby to turn head down with one day of Forward-leaning Inversions (FLI) in the window of 30–34 weeks. FLI has been successful even at 40 weeks or later. SpinningBabies.com's Transverse (Sideways) and FLI pages have safety tips and warnings to read first. A transverse baby may turn in a day.

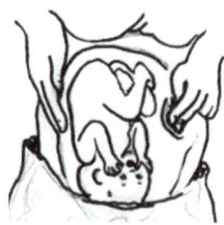

Once Baby Turns to a Vertical Lie
You will feel softness on the sides and firmness up through the middle when baby is either head down or breech. One side will likely be firmer, and so will the top of the womb. The head might already be too deep to feel easily. Most babies turn head down. If your baby turns breech, continue other techniques (page 62).

References
1. Jensen, J. G. (1992). Uterine torsion in pregnancy. *Acta obstetricia et gynecologica Scandinavica*, 71(4), 260-265. https://doi.org/10.3109/00016349209021049
2. Matthews, L., & Rankin, J. (2024). Muscle–the pelvic floor and the uterus. In J. Rankin (Ed.), *Physiology in Childbearing*. 5th ed., Elsevier, p. 297.
3. Webster, J. C. (1893). The occurrence and significance of rotation of the uterus. *Transactions of the Edinburgh Obstetrical Society*, 18, 149.

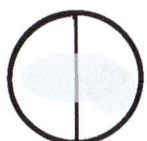 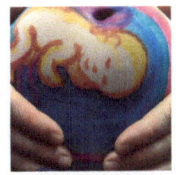 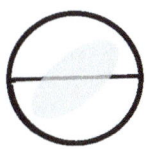 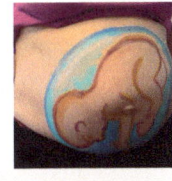 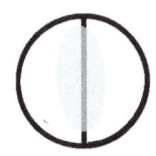 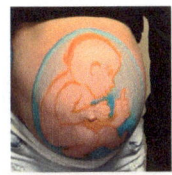

Head and Buttocks
The head is across from the buttocks.

Which Direction?
Is baby lying vertically, sideways, or diagonally?

It's Not a Lie
The direction a baby's body is lying is called *lie*.

Figuring Out What You Feel

Where do you feel the soft and firm parts of your uterus?

Which direction is baby lying in? Vertical, sideways, diagonal?

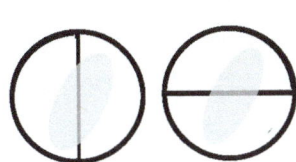 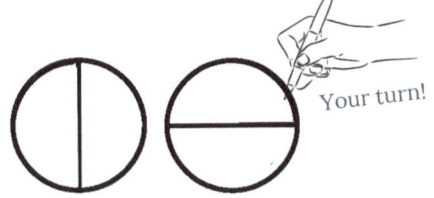 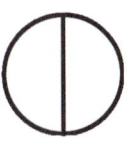

Your turn! Now make a shape to show the direction that your baby lies inside your belly.

Which Side Is Baby's Back or Baby's Front?

Next, find the back of the baby. The back feels smooth and firm, compared to lumpy. Baby's front is opposite the back. Kicks and wiggles are in the front of baby. Baby's legs and arms can stretch outward in front of baby. Knees can poke in front, and legs can stretch across your uterus to raise a foot on the other side.

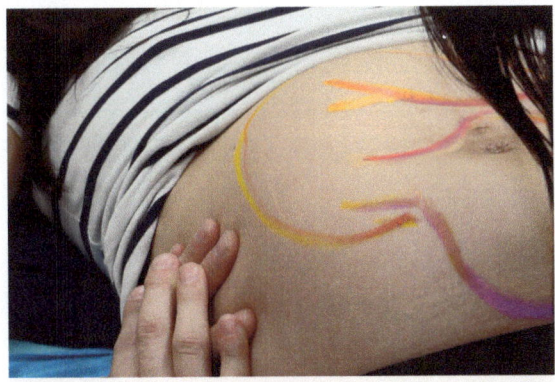 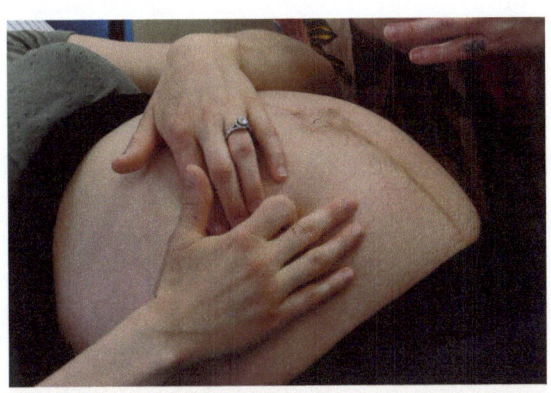

Back　　　　　　　　　　**Front**

Are Those Little Parts the Hands Fluttering or the Feet Kicking?

A delighted look of comprehension brightens a parent's face when they realize that the little lump they've been feeling is a foot! The smaller parts you feel are hands, feet, and limbs, with the elbows and knees. We call all of these "small parts."

How can you tell what parts are feet and hands? Taps with a random rhythm are often from hands or feet. Rhythmic taps may be hiccups. Feet press more firmly than hands. During baby's rest, hands and feet don't move much and are not felt.

Feet

Feet may be felt kicking several times a day. Feet kick outward in play, during crying, and when baby is startled. (Don't let people startle your baby to see if they can, as the adrenaline jolt teaches baby to feel unsafe with them.)

When the legs bend at the knees, the feet are close to baby's pelvis. When the legs stretch out, the feet push away from the buttocks, even across the womb. Two feet pushing out together can make a bulge the size of a bum!

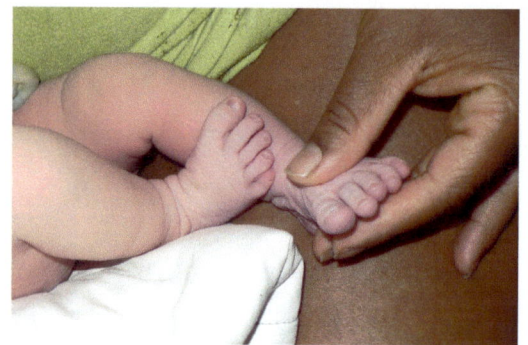

When marking, we'll use K's for kicks (feet) and W's for wiggles (hands).

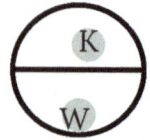 Hands and feet may be on opposite sides or the same side.

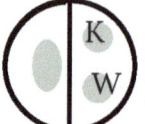 Knees bend and bring the feet close to baby's bottom.

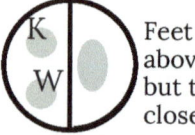 Feet may be far above the hands, but they might be close together.

Hands and Feet
By 28-30 weeks, feet are usually above the navel; hands below.

Back Is Opposite
Hands and feet are opposite baby's back when baby faces a hip.

Together?
Though hands are mapped, the hands may not be felt very often.

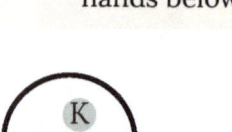

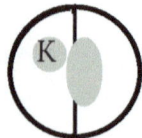

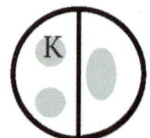

Strength
Feet can push out. Hands usually flutter and do not push out.

No Hands Are Felt
When baby's back is toward the front, the hands are not felt.

Back and Limbs
Hand flutters are not felt as often as feet kicks.

Hands

Small wiggles or flutters may be hands, especially near baby's head. Feet push; hands tickle. Don't worry if you don't feel baby's hands. Only certain baby positions allow a hand to reach your abdomen, where your body can feel them.

Hands, if felt at all, feel like tickles. Baby learns through touch and taste. Ultrasounds have shown baby's fingers rise to explore the mouth, cord, and genitals; tug an earlobe; or cover the eyes. Hands are often near the mouth, ears, and face. If you can actually feel a hand, you'll feel knuckles or fingers!

You may not feel baby's hands when:
- Baby's tummy and hands are turned toward your spine.
- The abdomen is less sensitive or is "padded."
- The placenta is low in front.

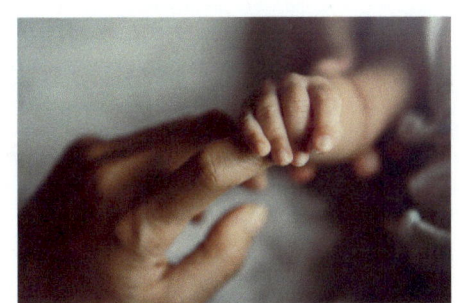

If the placenta covers the feet but not the hands, feel for more clues to see if "feet" are really hands.

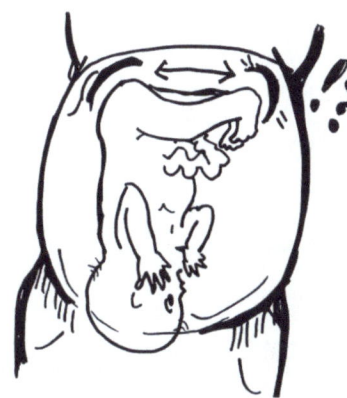

When a head-down baby stretches their legs, the buttocks will bulge outward on the opposite side of the feet. During baby's stretch, the womb seems to become triangular. There's a bulge on both sides!

I've been asked, "Could my baby have two heads?" No, it's just that both feet are pressing out on one side while baby's bum (buttocks) is pushing out on the other. The head is down by the pubic bone, nowhere near these bulges. Recall if your care provider mentioned where baby's head is located.

What Do You Feel?

Where do you feel baby's kicks? Which side? Top or bottom? Put a K there. Is your baby positioned so you can feel their hands wiggle? Put a W there.

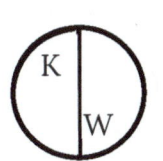 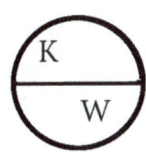 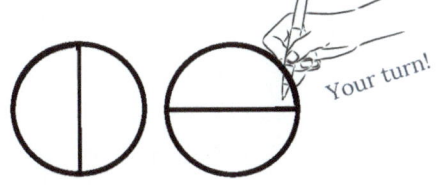

Now put K's for kicks and W's for wiggles where you feel your baby's feet and hands.

How Can I Find Baby's Legs and Arms?

You may be able to feel a thigh, leg, or knee. When baby is head up and facing the side or front, you may feel an arm.

A baby's leg or arm feels like a cylinder. A small bump near the end of a cylinder is a foot, while a small bump in the middle is a knee or elbow!

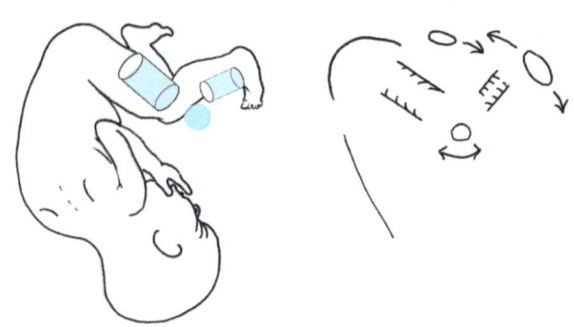

See the drawing here to help you visualize how legs can make cylinder shapes. Notice the cylinder coming out of the bulge made by baby's bum. Where you feel kicks will change when knees bend or baby turns. The feet can arc along an entire quadrant or cross into another quadrant. No big kicks? Feet may be close to the trunk. If the placenta covers the feet, you'll only see a rise of the belly.

Arms can feel like cylinders too. Arms are smaller than legs. If the head has a cylinder near it (an arm), it will not connect to the head like a thigh connects to the hip. When baby is head down, it's unusual to feel arms. Follow the cylinder-shaped limb to the other end for a clue about which limb it is, if you can.

Arms are not often close enough to the abdominal wall to feel. You might be able to feel the arm near the head of a baby in a breech position. Don't be concerned if you can't feel "cylinders."

Knees and elbows feel similar. When baby faces forward, you may see knees sliding past your navel. Knees and elbows feel like small, hard balls.

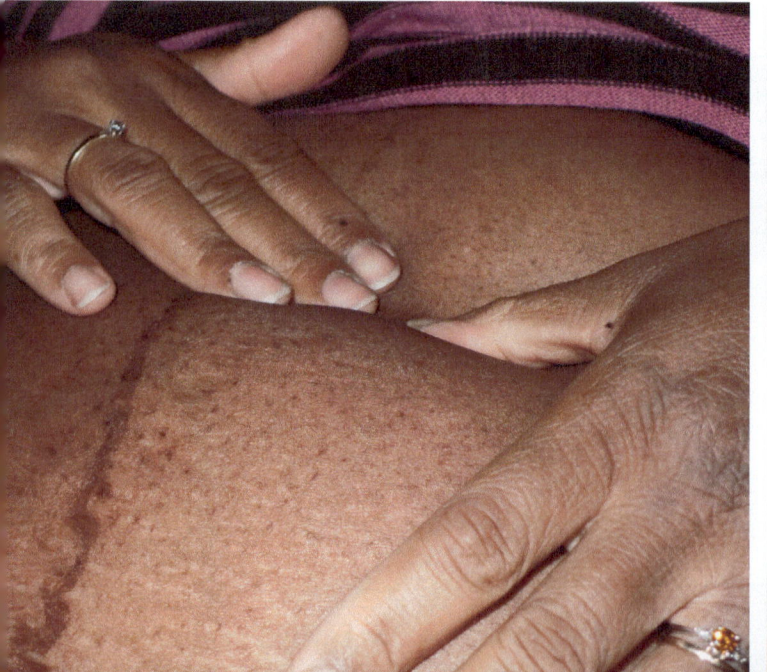
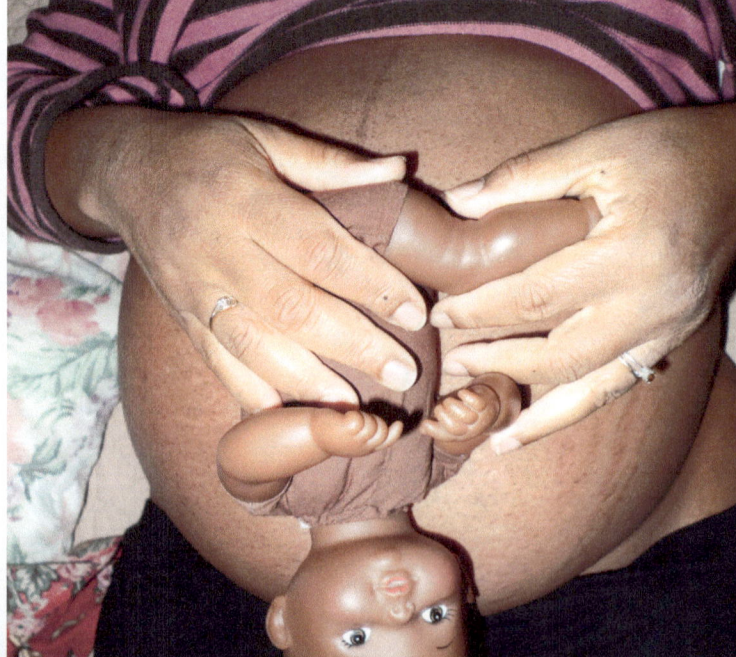

Finding Baby's Head

Baby's head will be somewhere along the outer edge of your womb by late pregnancy. As your uterus grows to reach your ribs, a head or bum will be farther from the navel. The head is easier to find if it is up than if it is already down.

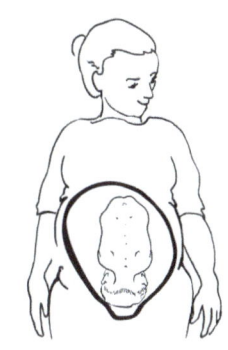

As you search, let your belly relax while you go slow to allow your fingers to pass the muscle layer. Before 36 weeks, for a head-down baby, search at or just above your pubic bone. Press deeper beneath the bone (closer to your spine) in the last month.

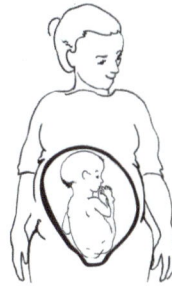

When baby is head up, the head is usually easy to find in the fundus, near your ribs, and not likely near your navel. Check below the right ribs; if not there, then try the top left or top center. If you aren't sure if a bulge is baby's head or bum, repeat another night. Again, press your finger pads in slowly and deeply.

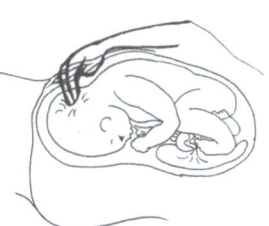

Once baby is both head down and low in the womb, you'll have to reach the depth of two finger joints just to find the curve of the back of baby's head. If the head is facing forward, baby's forehead is not so deep.

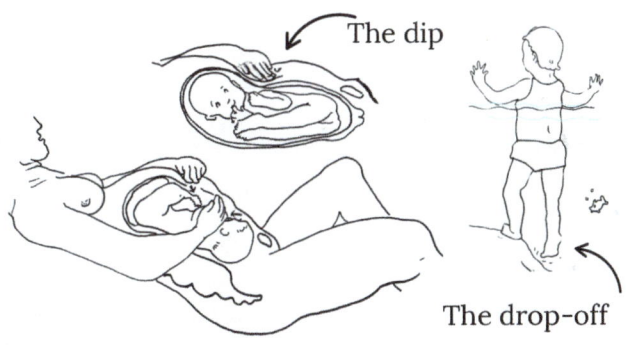

The dip

The drop-off

The neck makes a dip between baby's head and shoulder. Ever step off a drop-off at the beach?
Finding the dip by the neck is like finding a drop-off! Unlike the bum, which has no dip, this dip is a clue that this bulge is a head.

 Let's think about this: Touching your baby's head this way will not hurt baby. When you walk and change positions, baby's head will occasionally, gently bump your pubic bone, backbone, or ribs. Nature pads baby's head with your tissue layers and amniotic fluid.

Don't expect baby to be protected from the effects of bouncing fast while driving down a rutted road, though! Pressing with the pads of your fingers to contact the surface parts of baby is fine for baby.
Be confident that baby enjoys being stroked on the head and back.

Is Baby Facing Backward or Forward?

If your baby is facing backward (**an anterior position**), the firmness of the back and buttocks is wide across the front, centered or somewhat to the side.

A foot kicks up on one side; hands and knees will be tucked toward your back. With your baby's back in front, a care provider can find the heartbeat easily.

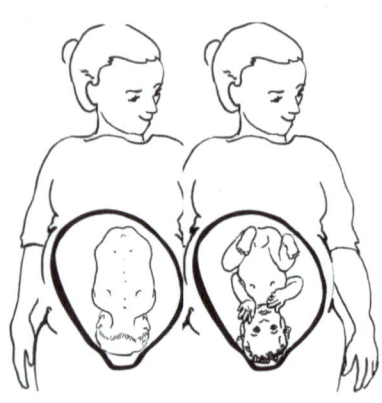

If your baby is facing forward (**a posterior position**), your baby's knees will be close to the surface. You may see a knee slide by or poke out near your navel. Feet will be close to the bum when knees are bent and stretch far from the bulge occasionally.

In fact, you may feel only feet and knees and not find a bulge if baby's bum is nearer your spine and can't be felt. Then, neither side of your belly will be fuller than the other. Baby's hands are in front, and you'll feel them playing.

Your care provider may search to find the heartbeat.

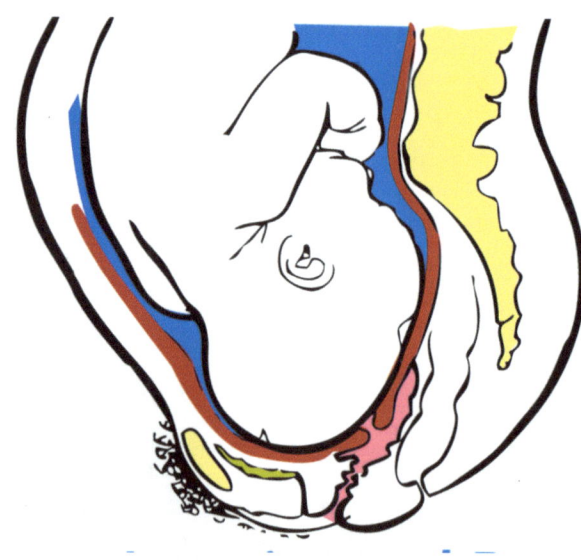

Direct Anterior Position (OA)

The OA baby may engage by 39 weeks. The symmetrical crown helps ripen the cervix. Hands aren't felt.

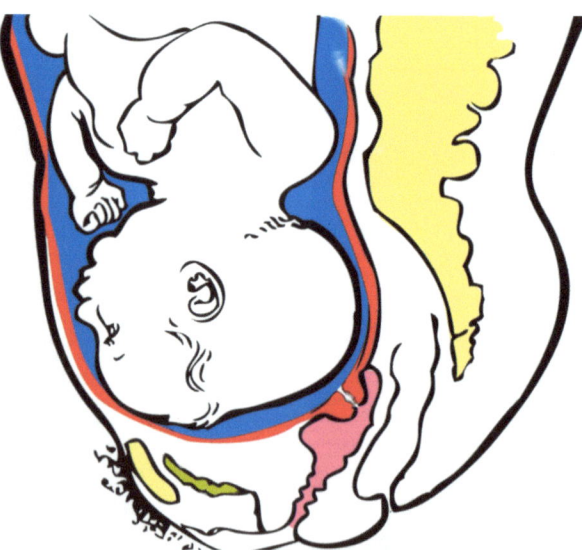

Direct Posterior Position (OP)

The OP baby may sit high and be slow to stimulate the cervix to thin out. Hands can be felt low on both sides.

Before You Draw a Map, Give Easy Answers

Your turn!

Date ___ ___ / ___ ___ / ___ ___

Today, I feel baby's small parts Y ☐ N ☐ .

I feel baby's small parts on my left ☐ , right ☐ , or both sides ☐ .

I feel them above ☐ , below ☐ , or both above and below my "navel line" ☐ .

Today, the biggest kicks are higher than the smaller flutters Y ☐ N ☐ .

I feel sure I felt the baby's back on the _____ side or front.
Left ☐ , Right ☐ , Front ☐ , Not sure or not found on this date ☐ .

I found the bulge at the side marked or center:
Left ☐ , Right ☐ , Center, above the navel ☐ .

I know my baby's head is up ☐ , down ☐ , to the side ☐ .

Date ___ ___ / ___ ___ / ___ ___

Today, I feel baby's small parts Y ☐ N ☐ .

I feel baby's small parts on my left ☐ , right ☐ , or both sides ☐ .

I feel them above ☐ , below ☐ , or both above and below my "navel line" ☐ .

Today, the biggest kicks are higher than the smaller flutters Y ☐ N ☐ .

I feel sure I felt the baby's back on the _____ side or front.
Left ☐ , Right ☐ , Front ☐ , Not sure or not found on this date ☐ .

I found the bulge at the side marked or center:
Left ☐ , Right ☐ , Center, above the navel ☐ .

I know my baby's head is up ☐ , down ☐ , to the side ☐ .

Download a printable PDF of this page. CLICK or SCAN ME

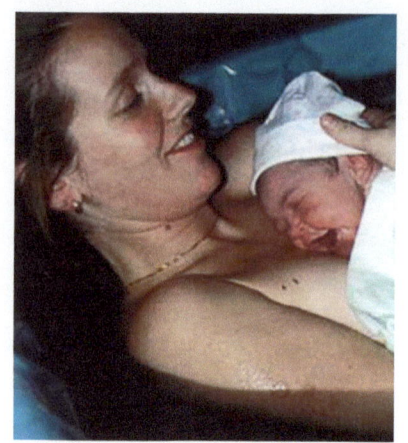

Katie's Using The Belly Mapping® Method

Katie is the inspiration for The Belly Mapping® Method. Shortly before the birth of her second child, she wondered if her baby was coming into her pelvis in a posterior position, facing the front. She knew some posterior births are challenging and was concerned. My reassurances fell flat, so I asked if I might draw her baby's actual position on her belly with her child's nontoxic markers.

Katie often felt kicks on the softer right side. Her baby's bottom was high on the left.

On Katie's map, a curved line shows where I felt the bulge on top. It matches baby's bum in my drawing on Katie's belly.

A line defines baby's back, while a curve below shows baby's head is partly in her pelvis.

A K is where baby kicked and a W is where Katie felt a hand when lying down.

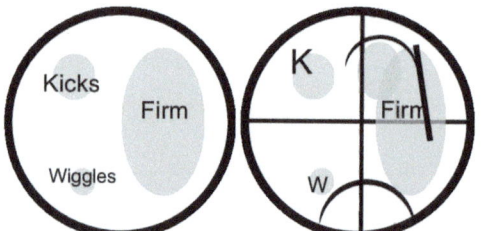

As Katie looked in the mirror (above right), she laughed—*and her labor began!* The proof of her baby's ideal position is in both their smiles just hours later (top).

Compare Katie's sensations and findings above to the posterior map below. Notice how many small parts move across the front. This was not a smooth, firm back. When the baby is posterior, the knees and hands create a lot of action up front.

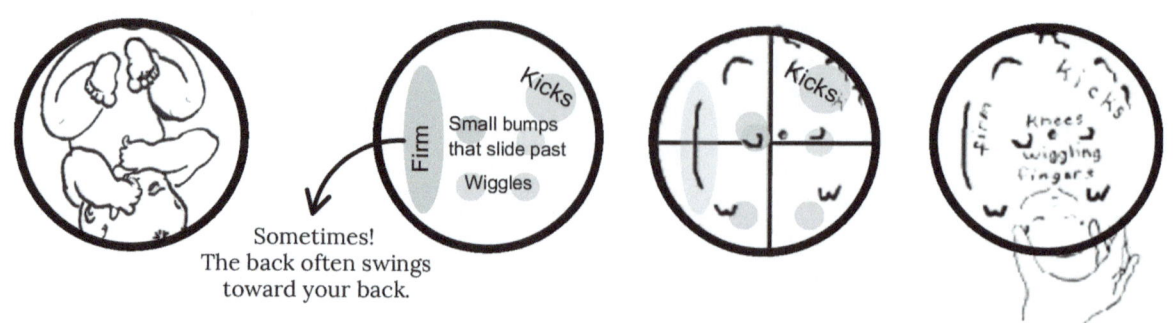

Your Turn

This template is for your first try. Scan to **download** and print a PDF.

These key questions are your primary guide to fill in your map.

1. Is one side of your baby harder, smoother?
Draw a line marking the outline of the edge of that firm, solid part of the baby.

2. Do you find a bulge at the top? The edge of your baby's body at the top? It may shift or slide occasionally, rising up. Where is it now?
Draw a curve there.

3. Where do you feel your baby's feet?
Put K's for the strongest kicks.

4. Where do you feel your baby's hands?
Write little W's on the exact location(s). Do they go near the dotted circle?

5. Can you remember where you or your care provider heard baby's heartbeat?
Draw a little heart on that location.

6. Do you know where your baby's head is?
Put a circle for the baby's head. The head may be under the dotted circle.

Try This Practice Map

Key to the Markings:

1. Draw a line for the firm, smooth back.
2. A curve for the bulge at the top.
3. A zigzag or letter K for a kick. You may have two areas for K's.
4. A W for a wiggle. Are there wiggles in the dotted circle?
5. Add a heart, if you know where it was heard.
6. If you find baby's head, make a circle there.

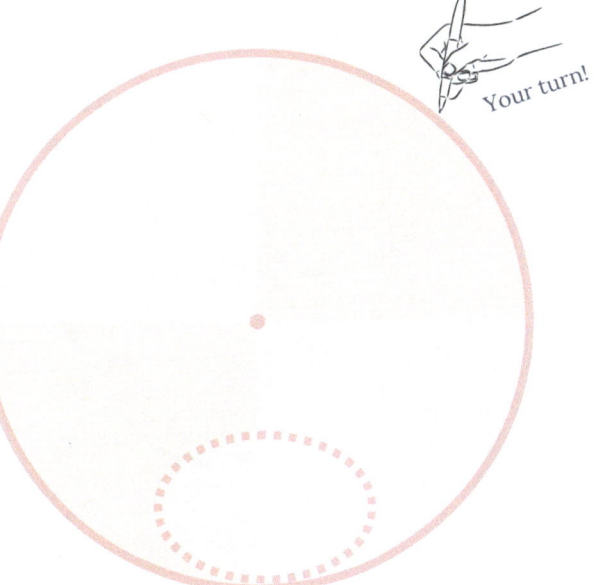

©2025 Spinning Babies®. All rights reserved. Spinning Babies® is protected by United States Trademark Nos. 4,200,336 and 5,527,742, and international trademark nos. 1,441,573 and 1,443,977. Spinning Babies® may not be used without permission.

Sensation Maps for The Belly Mapping® Method

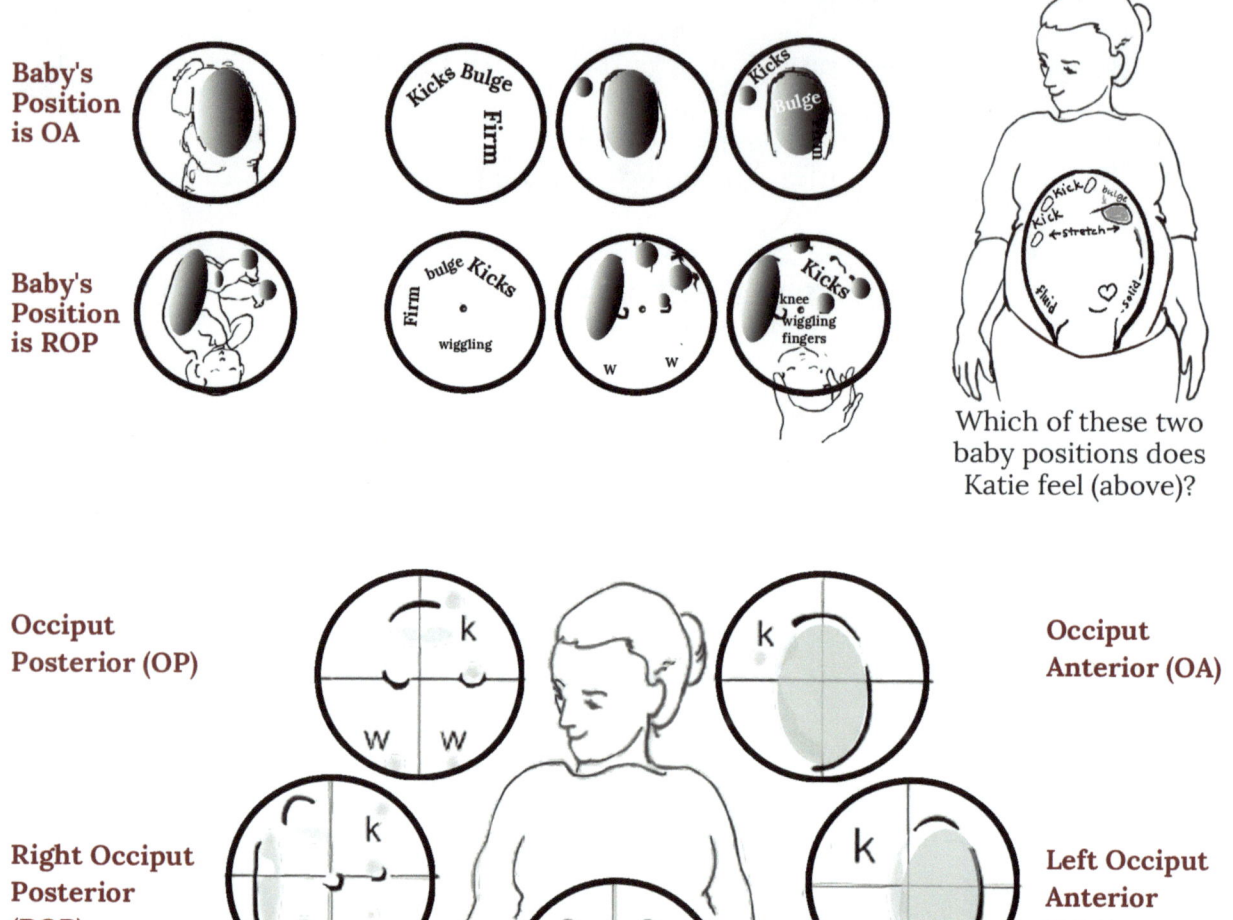

Which of these two baby positions does Katie feel (above)?

Using the quadrant system, you can map sensations and figure out the position.

26

Sensations Reveal Positions

Compare your answers on page 25 with the descriptions below. If baby changes position, you may notice more easily. Trust yourself. Once you feel confident, continue to the section on what to do.

If you find your baby is not head down, go to the breech section on page 53.

There are eight basic head-down **positions**. We begin with left-sided positions.

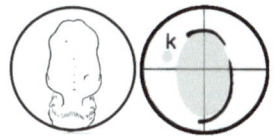

Occiput Anterior (OA)
Baby's back is firm in the front and center of your belly. Any kicking is up at the top or top right. Baby's bottom presses up in the top center or slightly left. The head is low and centered. Your care provider can easily hear baby's heartbeat across a wide area in the front. Both shoulders may be felt, but baby's right shoulder (on your right) will be a little closer to the surface.

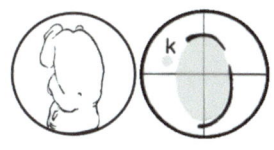

Left Occiput Anterior (LOA)
Baby's back is on your front left. Kicking is on the top right. Baby's bottom presses up in the top left or in the center. Baby's head is low, and you walk as if carrying around a ball (which you are!). Your care provider can easily hear the heartbeat left and center. The front shoulder is on the right of the center line. The main difference between OA and LOA is that the head is in a diagonal direction looking back to the right.

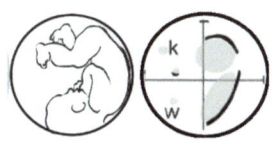

Left Occiput Transverse (LOT)
Baby's back and one shoulder are both on your left. Baby's hips shift left or right. The feet are far to the right, high or sometimes at navel level. A hand may wiggle on your lower right only occasionally, but not both hands at once. By 38 weeks, the head may be quite low, causing pressure twinges on your *cervix*. Your care provider can easily hear the baby's heartbeat toward the left.

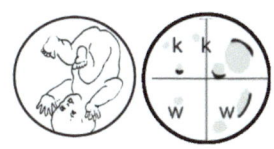

Left Occiput Posterior (LOP)
Baby's back is far over on your left. Baby's bottom makes a bulge in the upper left, sometimes shifting to the top center. You feel limb activity all over the front, mostly on your right. Baby's head may dip into the pelvis before the due date or stay high. The forehead can be found a little right of your center. Your care provider hears baby's heart on the far left.

Here are sensations of the right-sided head-down **positions**.

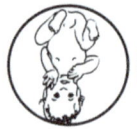 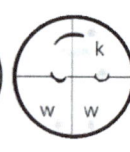

Occiput Posterior (OP)
Baby's back is along your lumbar spine, back-to-back. Kicking is across the top. Knees slide past the front in the last month or two. Baby's bottom occasionally presses up in the center. Baby's head is high, sometimes on or rubbing the pubic bone. Your care provider searches for the heartbeat, finally finding it far on the right. A shoulder is on the right, if found at all. Hands are felt low in front. The head may bump the bladder. Baby rarely engages without strong labor. Some OP babies will tuck their chins, but few engage before labor. A dip in your belly may show the dip between knees and chest. This isn't always noticeable, though it is considered a classic sign of OP.

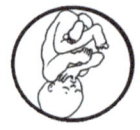 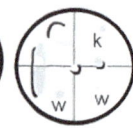

Right Occiput Posterior (ROP)
Baby's back is far to your right near your back. Kicking is on the top left. Baby's bottom presses up in the top right and occasionally in the center. Baby's knee or knees may sometimes slide across the front of your abdomen, past your navel. Baby's head tends to be high and may overlap the pubic bone. Your care provider searches for the heartbeat far to the right. The electronic fetal monitor easily slips away from the narrow range where the heartbeat can be heard and is often replaced.

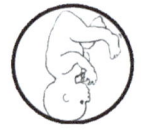 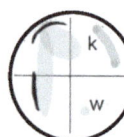

Right Occiput Transverse (ROT)
Baby's firm back is far to your right. Your womb feels softer on your left. Baby's bottom makes a bulge in the upper right and may shift to the front and then move to the right again. The firm back stays far to the right. You feel baby's hands and feet on the left side. Engagement happens after consistent, strong contractions. Your care provider hears baby's heart on the right and may need to search to find it.

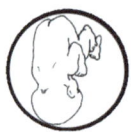 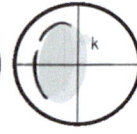

Right Occiput Anterior (ROA)
Baby's back fills the front right. You feel feet only on the left. Your care provider hears the heartbeat easily on the right. This position can be misdiagnosed when abdominal muscles or the broad ligament are overly firm (tight). No hands are felt.

Sensations Near the Bladder

A clue to which way baby is facing can be found near your bladder. In a head-down baby, wiggles between the pubic bone and navel are likely the baby's hands. If baby is head up, the feet may kick or slide past the bladder. Either way, a rule of thumb is that if you feel little wiggles on both sides of your center line, your baby is facing forward. Wiggles on only one side mean baby may be facing that side.

Many women feel no wiggles in the lower front of the abdomen. Feeling no sensation here is normal when baby is facing your back. Remember, an anterior placenta may hide the hands of a baby facing the front.

Other sensations in this area could be pressure on the bladder; a forehead "grinding" on the pubic bone in a face-forward baby; the pubic bone itself shifting; or, if deep inside, the lacy pull or "zing" of **cervical ripening**.

Facing Facts

A baby in the womb won't naturally play with their hands behind them. So both hands wiggling in front means baby is facing your front. If this is your experience, read later about how to care for a *posterior position* in labor.

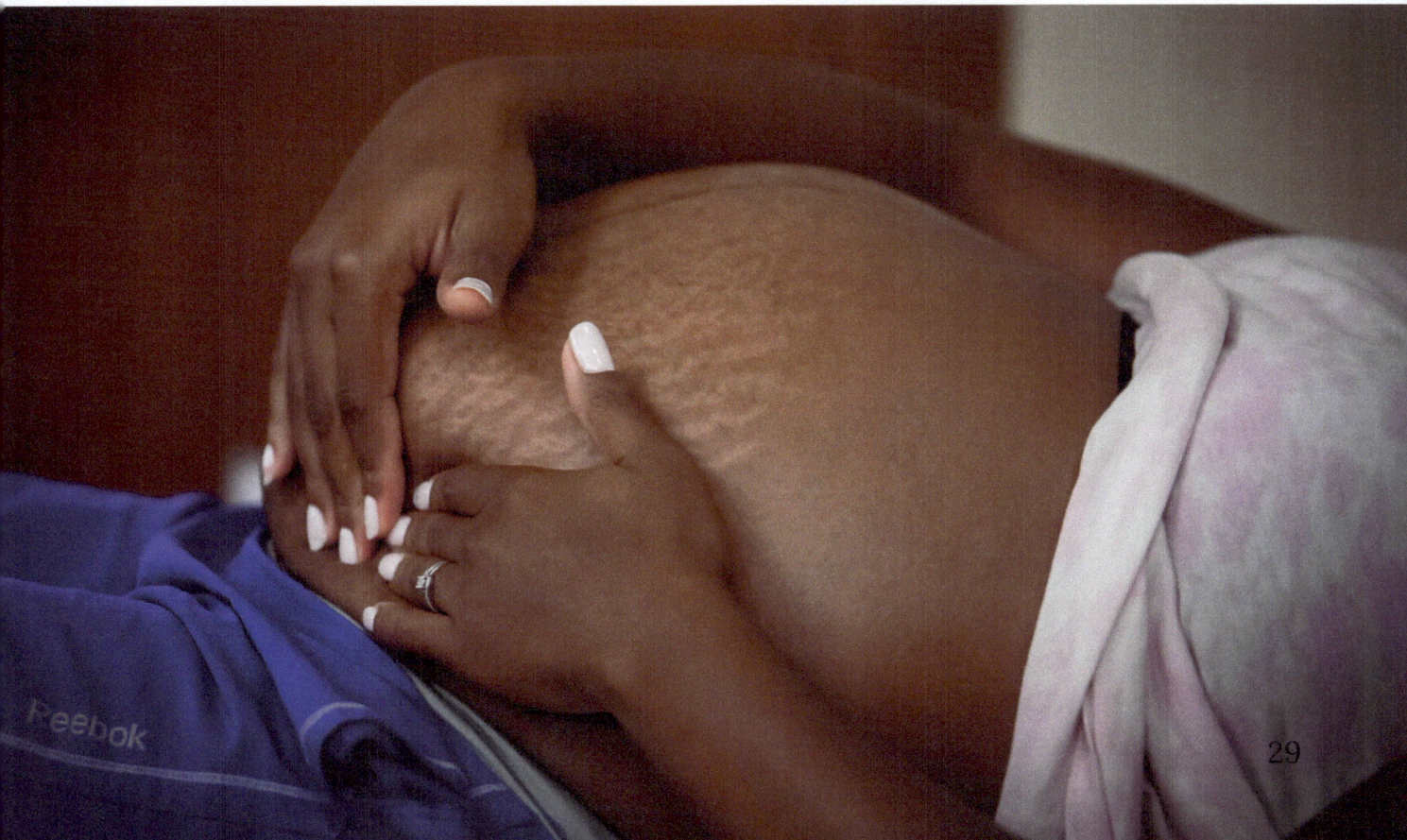

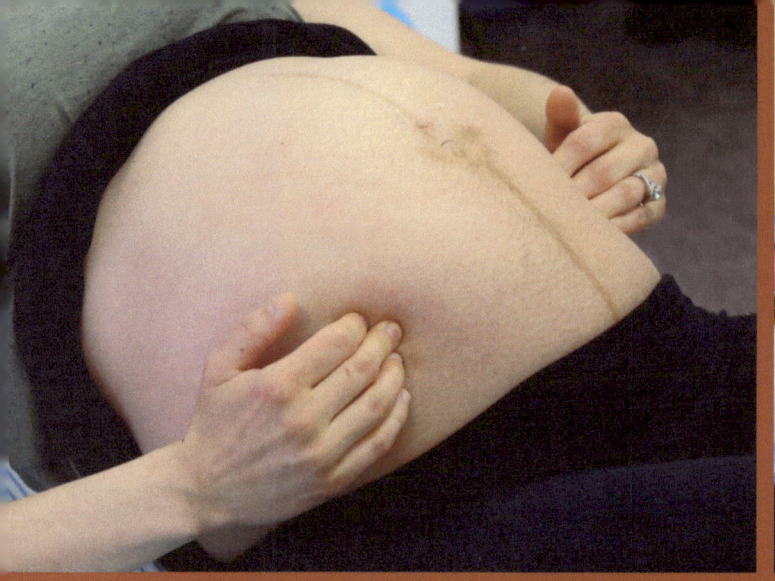
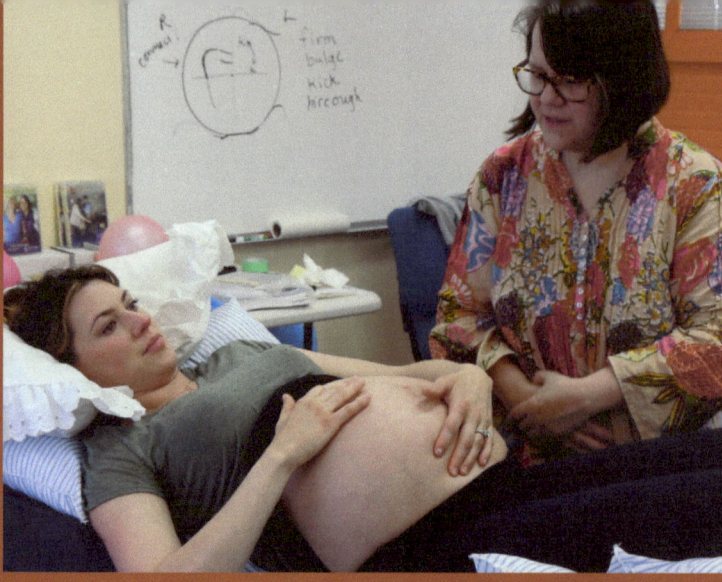
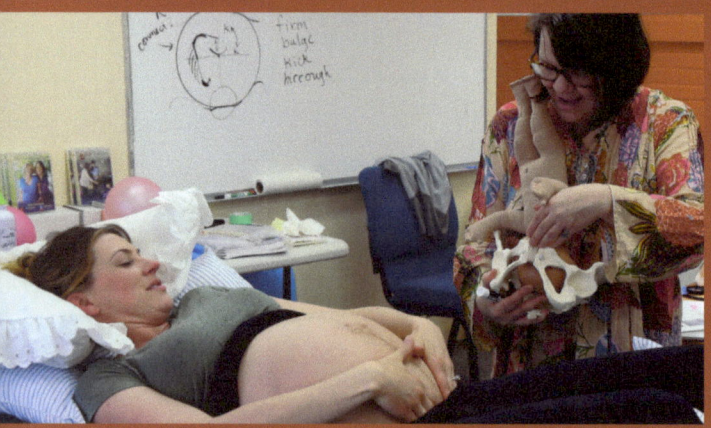
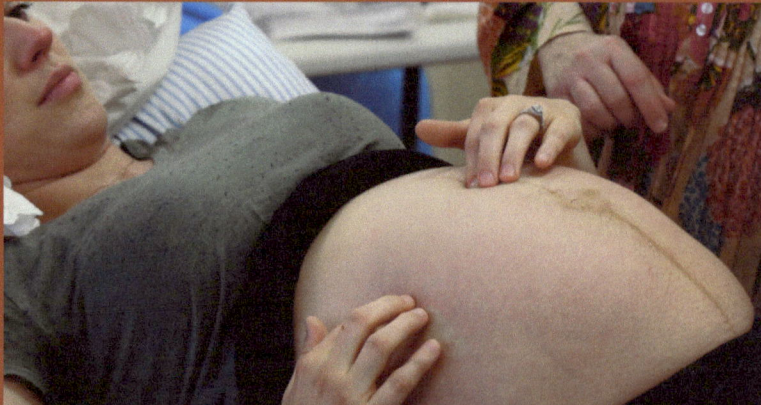
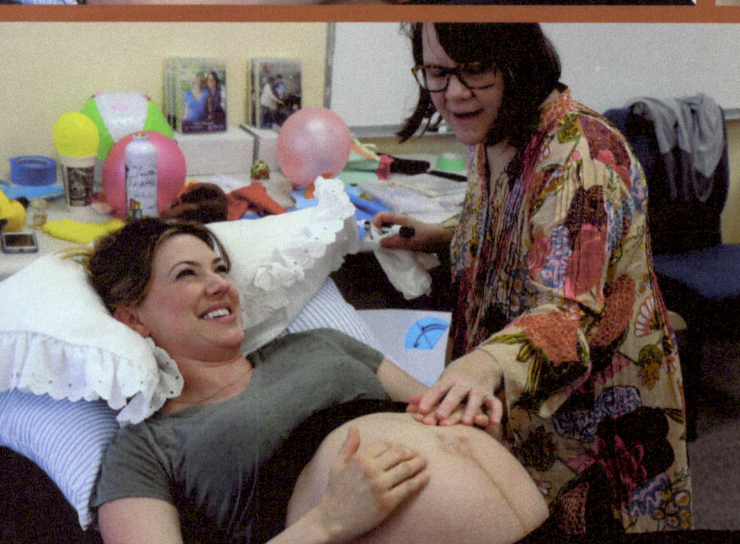
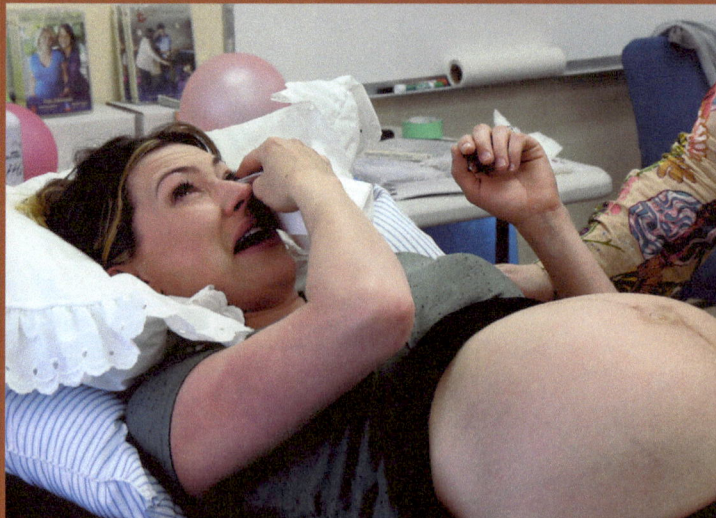

Deneé Tries The Belly Mapping® Method

Top row: 1. Deneé feels for the hard and soft sides. 2. Feeling the top and bottom.
Middle row: 3. Finding the head. 4. Is that a foot?
Bottom row: 5. Yes, that's baby's foot!
6. Deneé's love for her baby overflows with tears of joy.

Frequently Asked Questions

Now that you've made a map of your baby's general position, you may wish to skip to Step 2: Visualizing Your Baby (see page 37). Some of you may have more questions about what you're feeling. You can also bring this book to your *caregiver* for help with details.

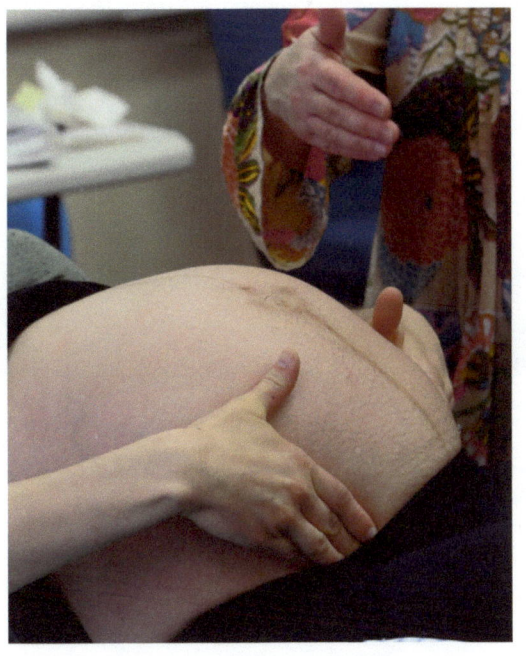

How Can I Find My Baby's Head?
We touched on the basics of finding the head on page 21. Most often, you will find your baby's head protected deep under your pubic bone. If you can't find it, check toward your hips. Otherwise, you may not be feeling deep enough. In pregnancy, your uterus will be softer; your fingers will be able to go in deeper to find the head. Press into your skin to the depth of half of your finger's length.

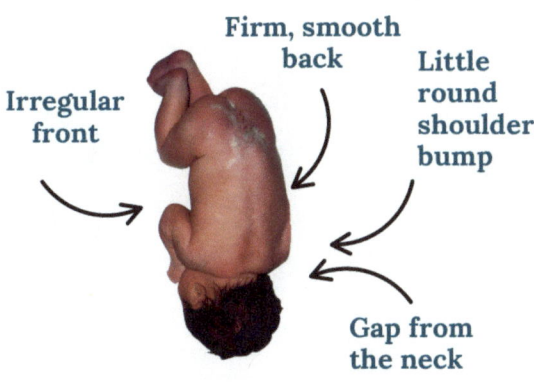

Baby's firm back ends with the shoulder. A shoulder feels like a small round corner near, but not touching, the head.

There is a small gap between the round corner of the shoulder and the head.

By the due date, the head may be so low in the pelvis that you can only feel the neck!

Is That a Head or a Bum?
The buttocks and head make similar-sized bulges. So how do you tell them apart? A cylinder shape, the thickness of two of your fingers, extends from the bottom and not the head. That cylinder is a leg. A cylinder near the head moves easily and does not lead to the bulge directly. That cylinder is an arm.
When baby faces the front, cylinder shapes by the pubic bone could be legs.

Will the Location of Hiccups Tell Me Where Baby's Head is?
Rhythmical taps for more than several seconds may be hiccups. Baby's hiccups are not a reliable indicator of being head up or down. Hiccups may be strongest near baby's back, but an echo might be heard farther away. If the hiccups change to the opposite side of your belly, it may mean baby did flip. Compare your clues!

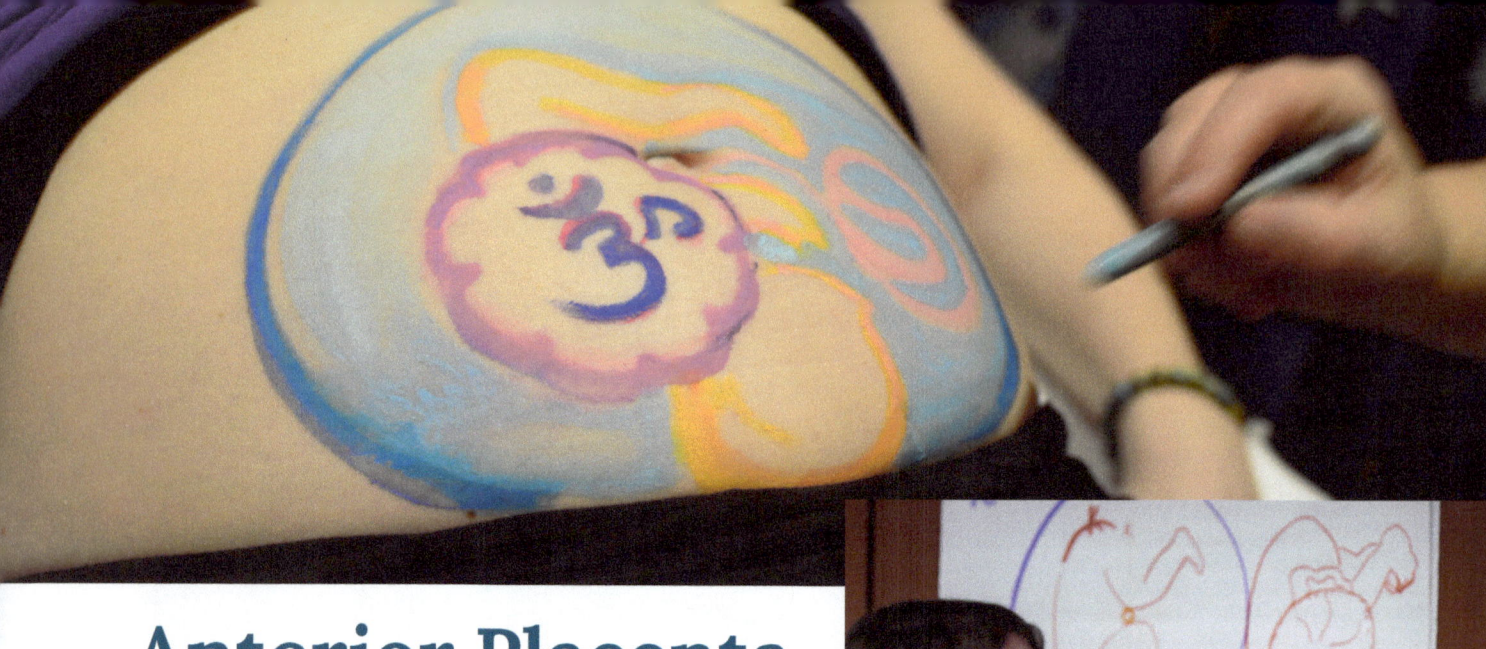

Anterior Placenta

The anterior placenta is located along the front of the uterus.

If you've had an ultrasound, you will have been told if your placenta is anterior. Check the summary of your scan. Baby will often face the placenta.

If you haven't had an ultrasound, you can guess. You might have an anterior placenta if:

- Feet poke out on the side, but you feel something fleshy, not hard, taking up much of the space in front.
- Baby is on the right side, but you don't feel hands, feet, or knees in front.
- Baby's movements make the womb rise in a general way, not with specific parts.
- This baby doesn't seem to move much or as much as a previous baby. **Call your care provider if baby's movement reduces from their usual habits.** Go have baby's movement evaluated now if you wonder.

Compare Two Maps

If you feel you might have an anterior placenta, draw one map with and one without a circle in the middle. Draw in the baby parts that may be beneath the placenta. Give yourself time to recheck another day. Repeating may reveal more details.

Tracking Baby's Position Changes

Compare your maps over time on this page. Taking time to make a series of maps can be a great help in **Step 2** (see page 37). The dates of your maps track position changes over time. Baby's position will not have changed significantly unless the back changes sides or head changes from top to bottom, for instance.

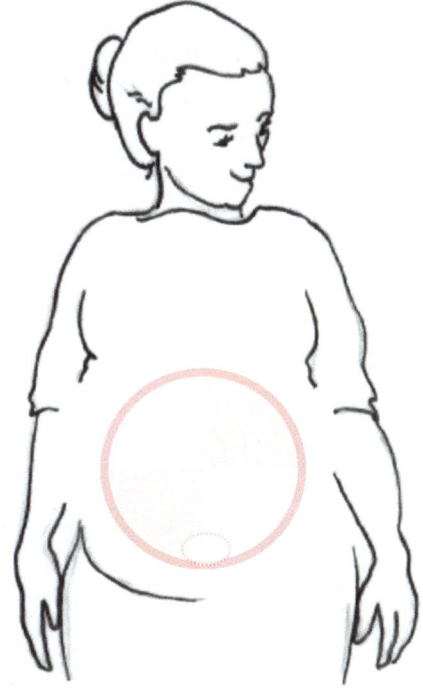

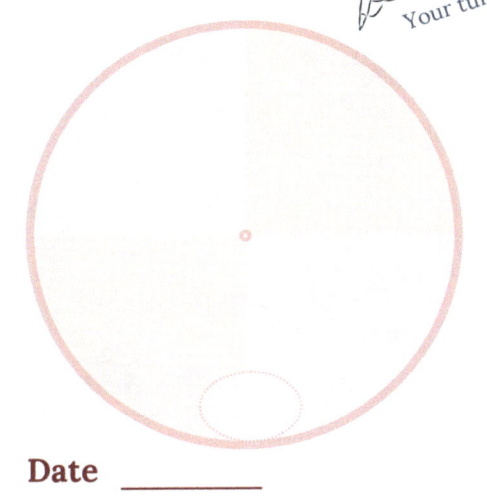

Date _____

Date _____

Step 1: Map the Kicks and Wiggles
1. Draw a line for the firm, smooth back.
2. A curve for the bulge at the top.
3. A zigzag or letter K for a kick.
4. A W for a wiggle (a softer "kick" area).
5. Place a heart in the area where you or your caregiver hears the baby's heartbeat.
6. Make a circle for the baby's head. Your caregiver can help you find the head.

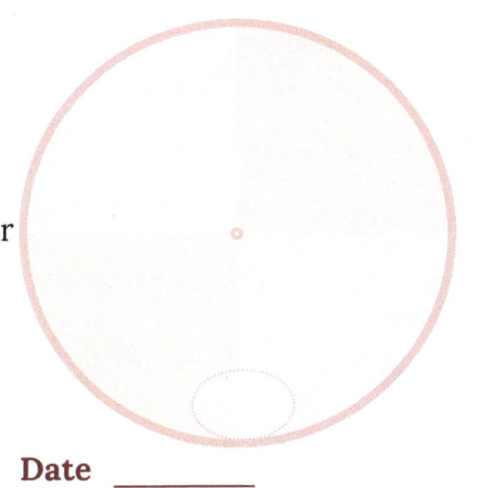

Date _____

©2025 Spinning Babies®. All rights reserved. Spinning Babies® is protected by United States Trademark Nos. 4,200,336 and 5,527,742, and international trademark nos. 1,441,573 and 1,443,977. Spinning Babies® may not be used without permission.

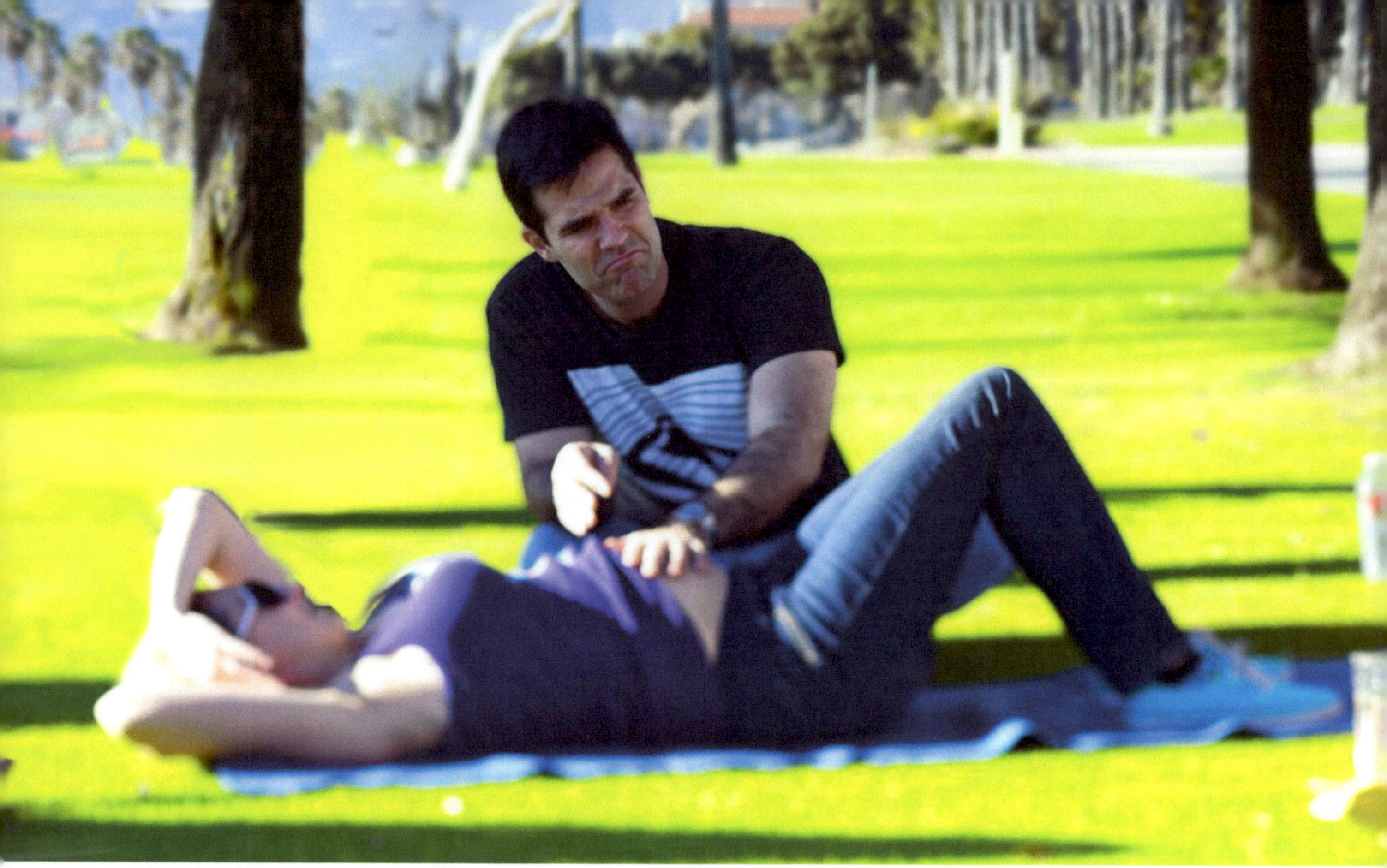

I Can't Find My Baby. What Can I Do?

When I can't tell a baby's position, I'll put my hand on the pregnant belly and call sweetly, "Baby, reveal yourself!" Wait. Six seconds later, a responding kick or shift shows another body part. And as baby gets larger, baby is easier to feel.

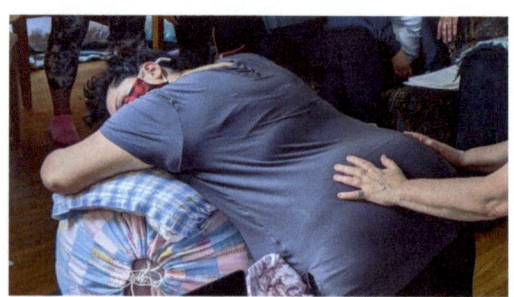

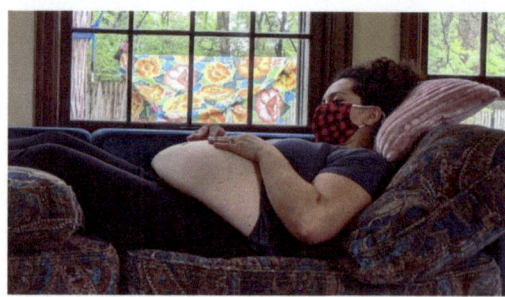

A Helpful Trick
If you or your care provider can't feel many details, one reason is that baby can slip deeper into your womb and away from the surface of your abdomen. If this happens, there is a trick:

Do slow pelvic tilts on hands and knees for three minutes to bring baby nearer the surface, then roll over very gently. Now feel. This won't work if you roll over too fast, because baby will be washed to the back of your womb.

Still can't find details in the third trimester? Could baby be behind the placenta? Page 32.

How Can I Tell If My Baby Changed Position?

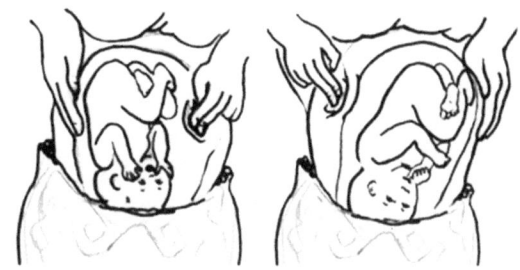
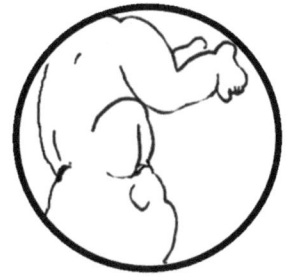
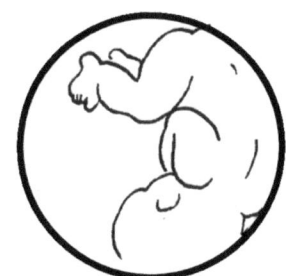

Confusion can occur when the womb slips to the side during sleep.

Let's say, before bed, baby's firm body is felt on the right. The left side is soft. Upon waking, the baby is now on the left. The left side of the womb is firm, and the right side is soft.

Did the baby switch sides?

After walking, though, baby "switched sides" again and is back on the right side. Is baby switching sides?

The baby may not be changing positions. The womb may be switching which side it is leaning toward.

The key is to know whether the kicks stay on the left side or change to the right. Kicks change location when baby's position actually changes.

Wishful Thinking

Even caregivers can misinterpret babies' positions. A common mistake is to confuse a little forehead for the nape of the neck. The assumption is that the baby is anterior when the baby is actually posterior. Look for several clues before assuming a baby's position. Is a knee sliding near the navel? Do hands wiggle on both sides of the center line? A hand in front is a strong clue baby is posterior. Babies play with their hands by their mouths, not behind their backs!

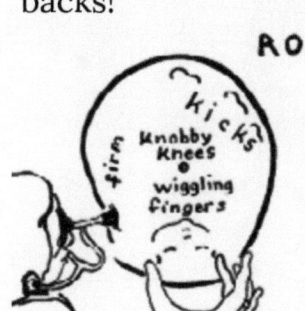
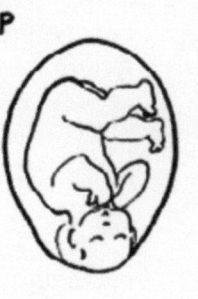
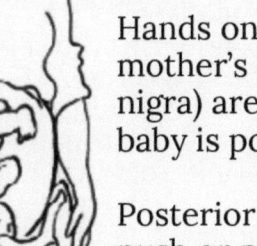

Hands on both sides of a mother's center line (linea nigra) are a sign that a baby is posterior.

Posterior babies will often push or punch the fetoscope or Doppler away from their face.

35

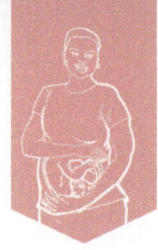

Embracing Creativity
The Science Behind Creativity and Pregnancy Wellness

Recent research involving 200 pregnant women in their second and third trimesters revealed a remarkable finding: Women with higher emotional creativity experienced significantly lower levels of pregnancy anxiety. This isn't just correlation—it suggests that developing your creative emotional skills can actively help you feel calmer and more confident during pregnancy.

The study found that when pregnant women were better able to creatively express their emotions, they experienced less worry about childbirth. They had fewer concerns about their baby's health, reduced anxiety about relationship changes, and greater overall emotional stability.

Why Emotional Creativity Matters During Pregnancy

Pregnancy is one of life's most transformative experiences, involving profound physical, psychological, and social changes. Your changing emotions during this time are your psyche's way of processing one of the biggest transitions you'll ever experience. The emotional skills you develop now will serve you well as you navigate the joys and challenges of parenting.

Three Practices to Develop Emotional Creativity

Emotional creativity can be cultivated through simple, enjoyable practices:

1. Keep a free-form journal. Write about your feelings and feel free to try different approaches. Create poems about your experience; draw or paint pictures that represent your emotions. Sing, dance, or act out what you are feeling. Make your own rules and ideas about what you feel like creating.
2. Collect images that inspire you that you will one day share with your child.
3. Surround yourself with art in a space that delights you every day.

Your Creative Journey Forward

Pregnancy is already one of the most creative acts possible—creating a new life. By exploring your own creative expression, you are actively developing skills that will enrich your entire parenting journey. You are creating your own unique language of love that you will simultaneously teach and learn with your family.

As you move through the remainder of your pregnancy, remember that every emotion you experience is valid and valuable. By approaching these feelings with curiosity and compassion for yourself, not only are you physically creating a person, but you are creating the environment for both your own well-being and your baby's healthy development. Your pregnancy is a unique story that only you can write. By embracing your unique perspective and ability to share it, you're ensuring that the story unfolds with greater joy, resilience, and connection.

Reference

Abbasmofrad, H. (2024). The relationship between emotional creativity and pregnancy anxiety in five to eight months pregnant women. *Journal of Modern Psychology*, 4(2), 19-26. https://doi.org/10.22034/jmp.2024.432708.1084

Step #2
Visualize Your Baby

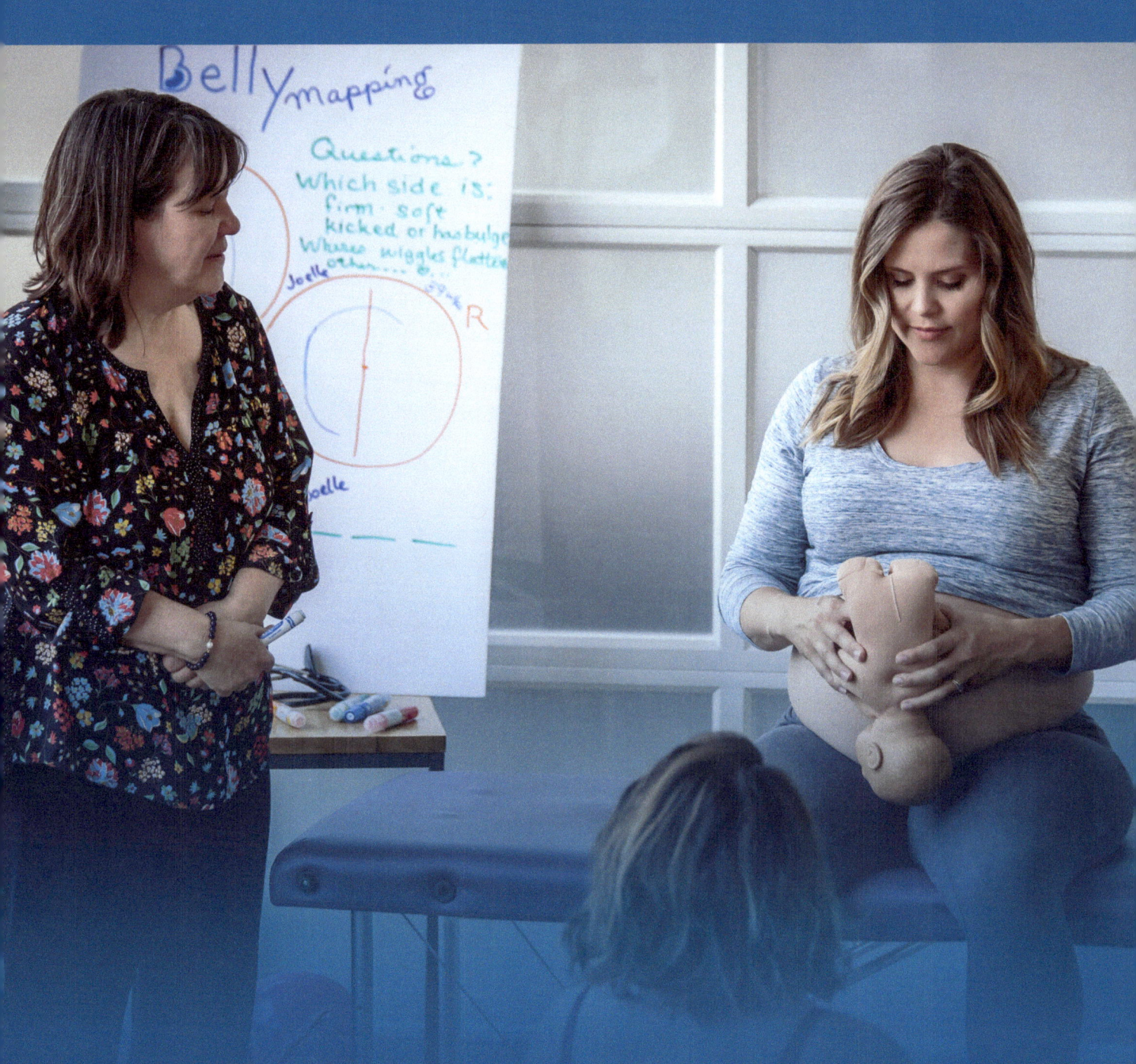

Step 2: Visualize Your Baby

Our minds need a three-dimensional version of a baby to understand more fully how a baby curls into the space inside. A doll will do the trick! Matching a doll's head and back to your map brings a sudden flash of insight into baby's bulges and bits. Step 2 creates more ease in imagining your real baby.

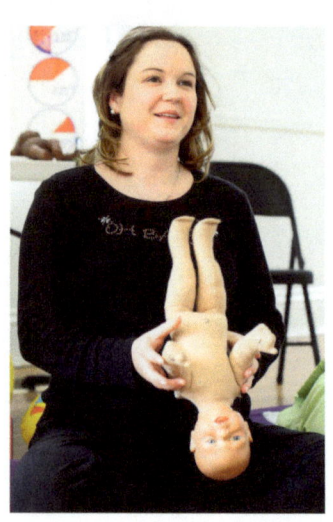

Get a doll or teddy bear about 12–20 inches (30–50 cm) long if you can. That's the length of a fetus at 30–40 weeks. Your doll may not be the same size as your baby, of course, and that's OK. Bendable arms and legs are easier to pose.

Positioning the Doll Over Your Map

Before positioning the doll over your belly, you may find your confidence grows if you arrange the doll over your map.

Match the head, feet, back, and buttocks to the markings you charted.

Accuracy is important if you are going to take action to help baby into a new position for your birth together. A general idea of how baby might be inside can also be enough.

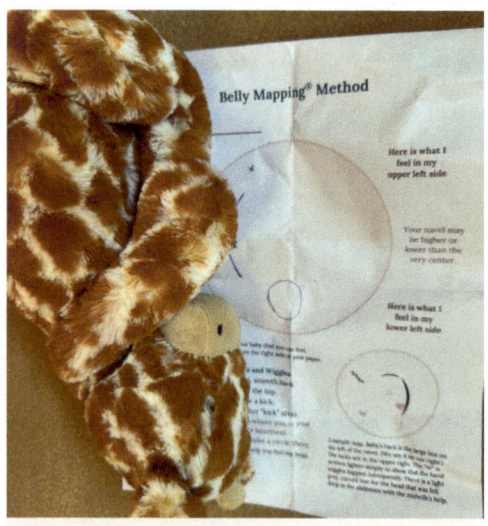

Joshua Giraffe in ROT

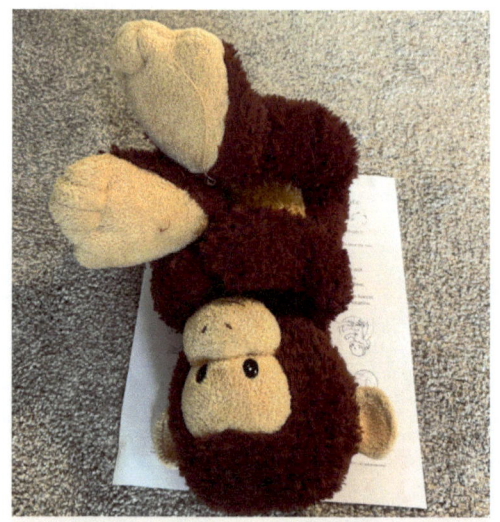

BoBo Shows us OP

38

Position the Doll Over Your Belly

With your map as your guide, position the doll's body parts (head, feet, back, and buttocks) over your belly. Put each doll part over the quadrant where you feel that part on your baby.

Remember that the left side of your belly is the right side of your map. And if you feel hands near your bladder, position the doll looking outward, like the photograph below.

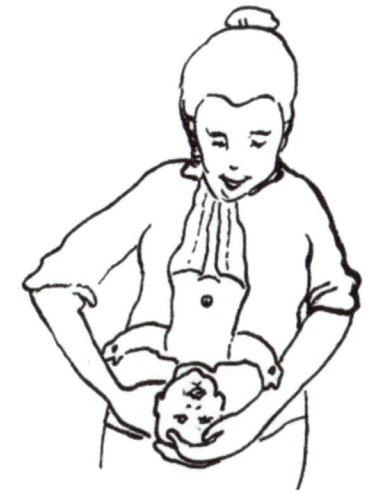

1. Start by putting them head-to-head.
Where did you draw your baby's head on your map?

Place the doll's head where you know your baby's head to be.

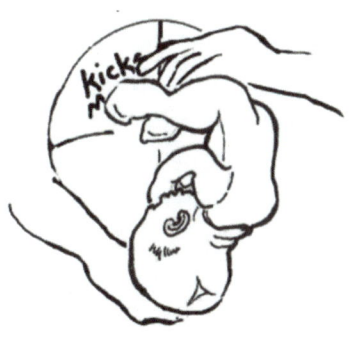

If your baby's head is down, the doll's head will likely be at or near your pubic bone, at the bottom of your abdomen, though some find baby's head nearer a hip.

2. Then, match hands and feet.
Without moving the doll's head, position the doll's feet so they are in the same place on you as they are on your map.

If you also feel wiggles near your pubic bone or navel, your baby's limbs are in front. Then you will need to turn your doll so its arms stick out in front of you.

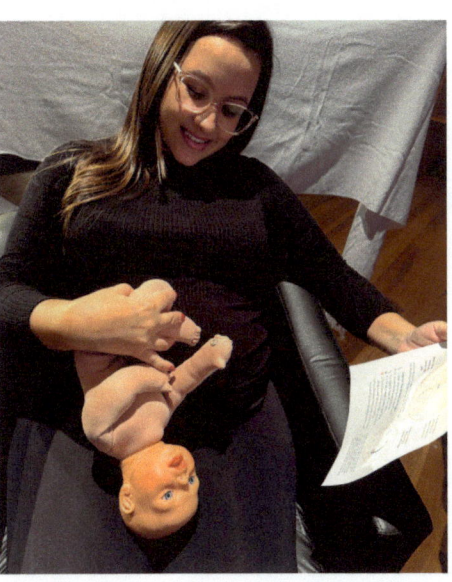

3. Match the doll's buttocks to the bulge.
Place the doll's buttocks so they correspond with the bulge you charted on your map.

Remember, you may have felt two bulges rise up when the baby's feet stretched. Use the consistent bulge for the doll's buttocks and keep the doll's feet where you usually feel them.

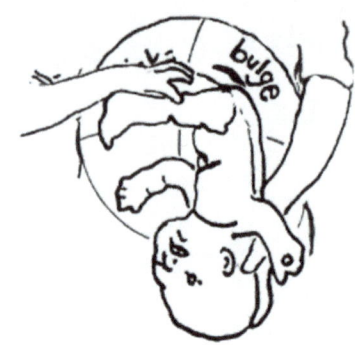

4. Lastly, match the backs of the doll and baby.
Without changing the position of the doll's head or feet, put the doll's back where it corresponds to the firm line you drew on your map.

It gets tricky if you didn't mark a firm back on your map. As explained in Step 1 (page 22), that means the baby's back is likely toward your own back. In that case, position the doll with feet and face forward, as described above.

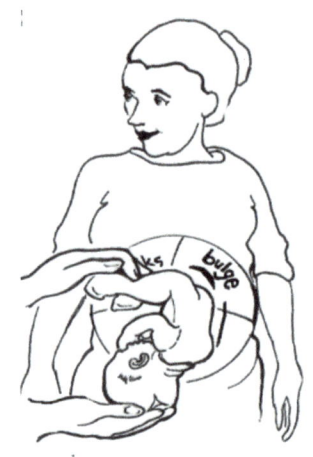

Up or Down?
If you still wonder whether your baby is head down or head up, take turns putting the doll's head in both places.

1. First, put the head down by your pubic bone, assuming your baby is head down, as most are. Does this put the feet, back, and butt in places that make sense according to your map?
2. Then, place the doll's head near the top of your womb, where you likely feel a bulge. Do baby's kicks, wiggles, and firm spots make more sense now, or less sense? Take your time.

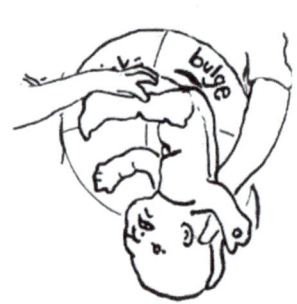

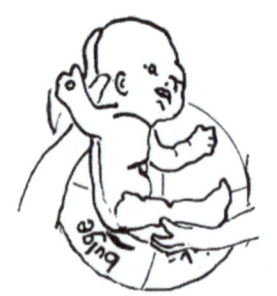

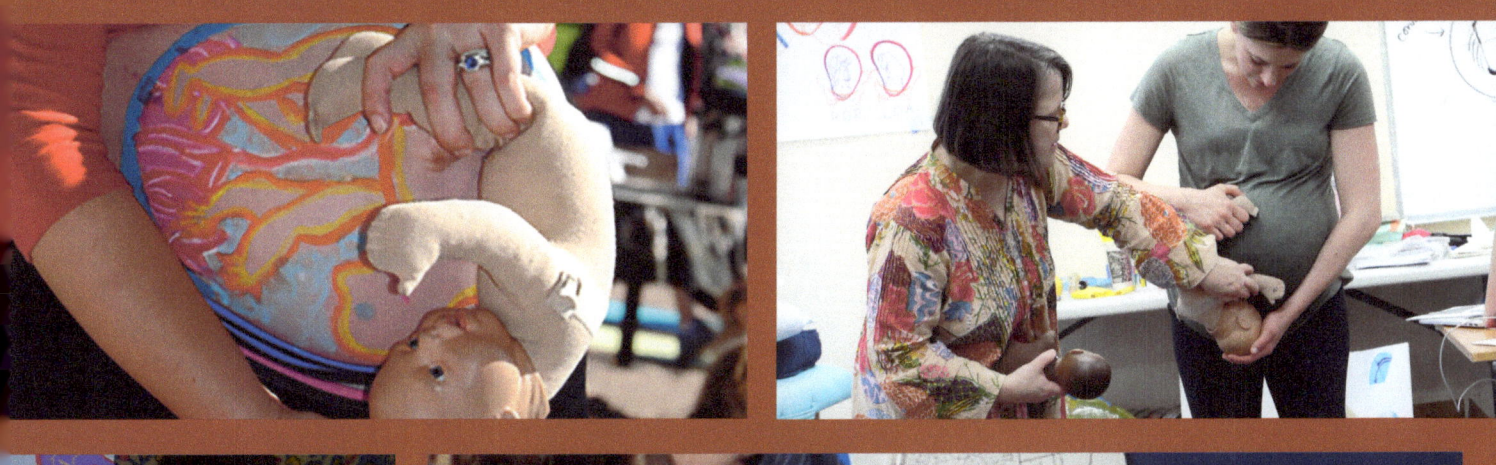
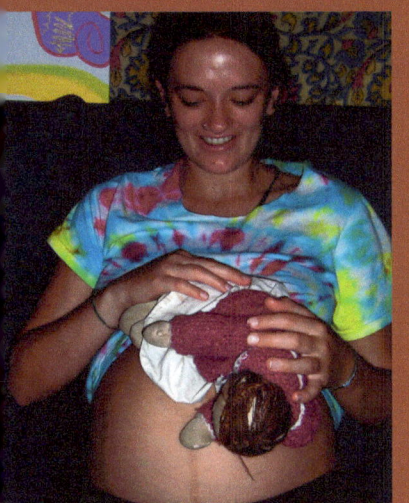
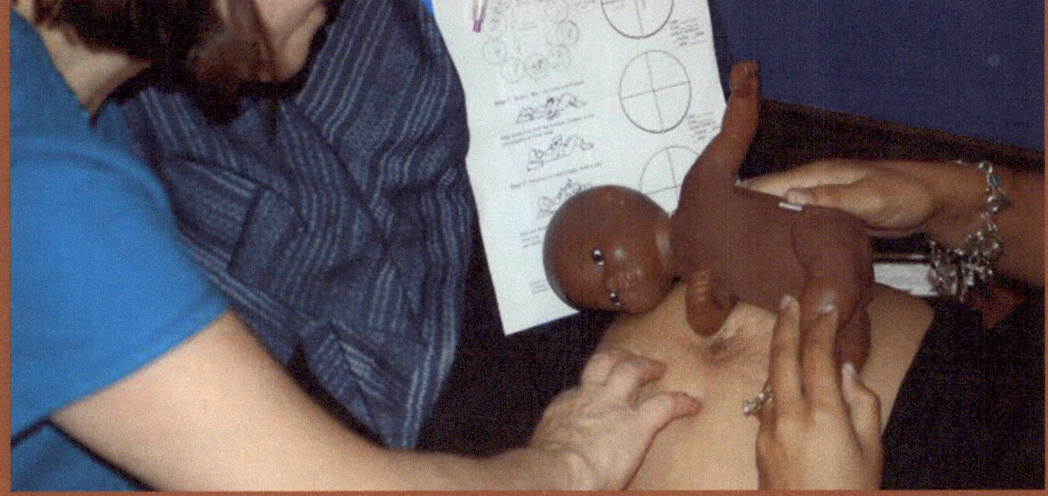

Parents Using a Doll to Visualize Baby's Position

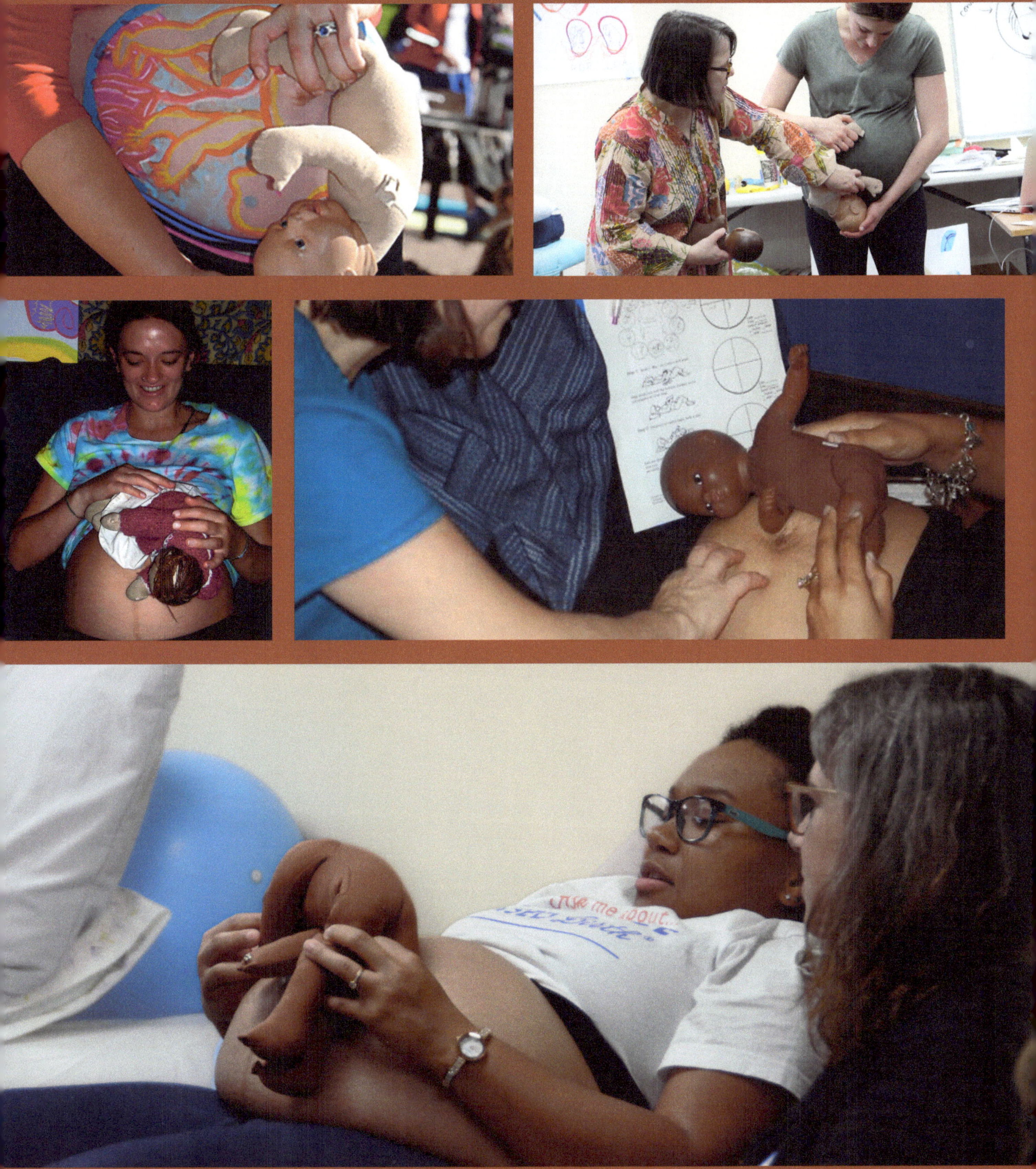

The Night The Belly Mapping® Method Was Proven

Dr. Bradford Bootstaylor and the sonographers of SeeBaby hosted an evening of The Belly Mapping® Method. To see for themselves, SeeBaby invited pregnant couples to compare their maps made using The Belly Mapping® Method with an optional and free ultrasound image.

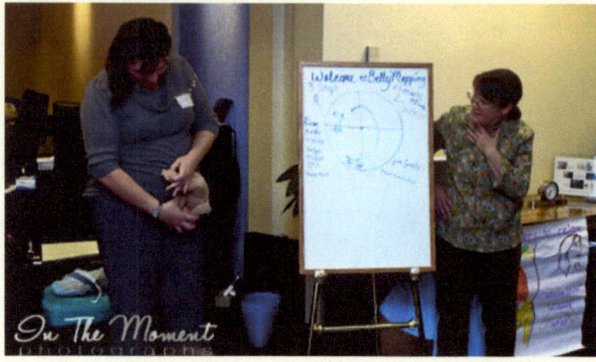
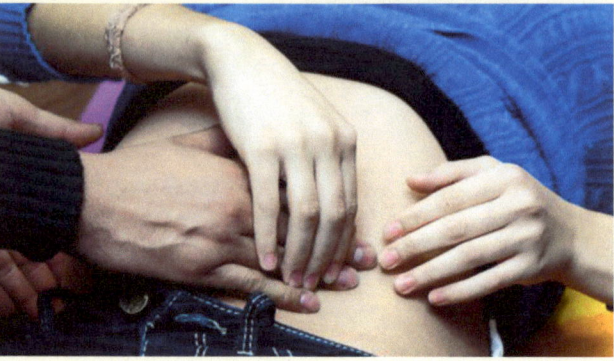

The evening was arranged by the Doulas of Georgia Birth Network, with photos by In The Moment Photography.

Five near-term women mapped their babies. Four of the five maps matched the scan with high accuracy. One woman, 24 weeks pregnant, wasn't able to map her baby's position, since I had forgotten to describe babies who are sideways in a transverse lie.

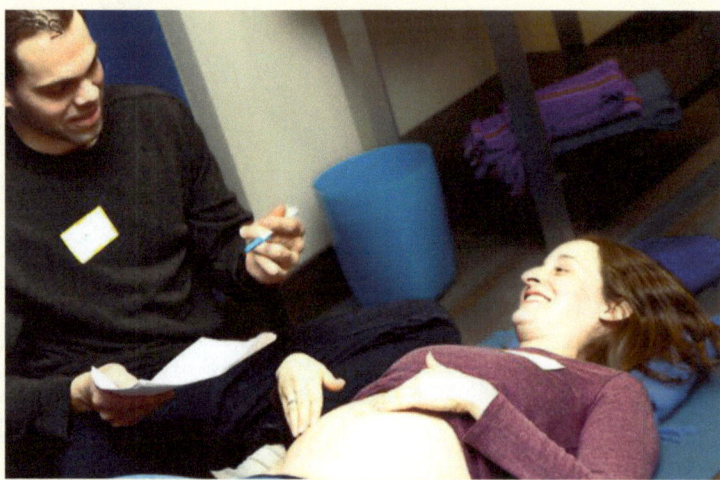

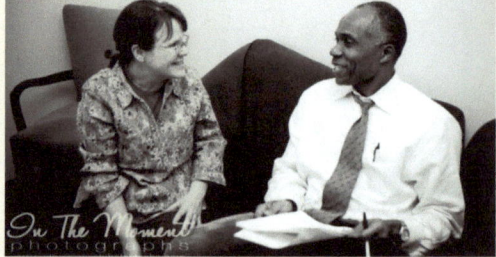

Above: Gail Tully and Dr. Brad Bootstaylor enjoy seeing the proof of the parents' abilities.

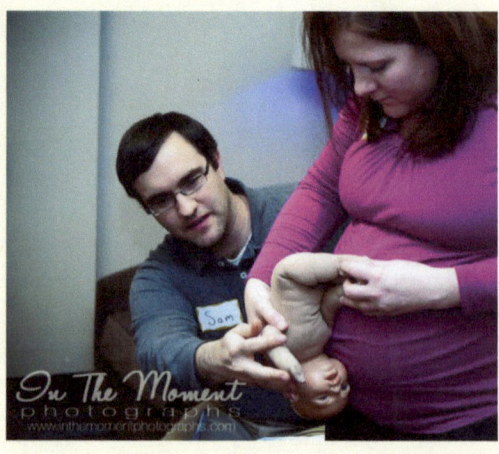

Above left: A mother demonstrates Steps 1 & 2. We see a map marked with her baby's kicks, wiggles, and bulges in four quadrants. She has put the doll's head down and moved the doll's feet into the upper right.

Top right and bottom left: Partners work together to map their babies' contours.

Bottom right: The partner offers a third hand to show baby's hand by their face. This matches the flutters she has been feeling by her bladder.

Dr. Bootstaylor and his team are amazed by the parents' ability to map their babies' positions.

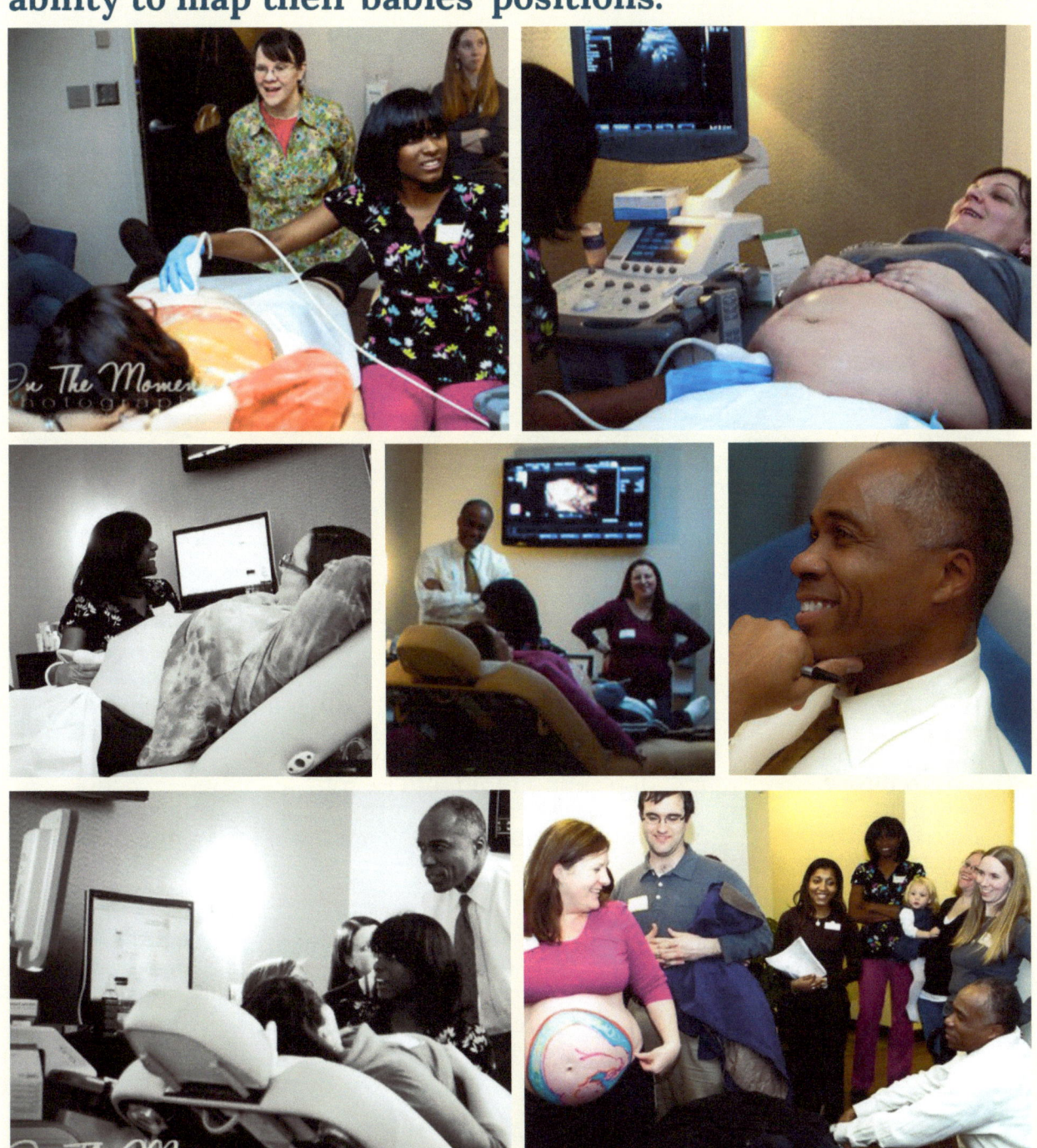

Top two rows: Photos show the delight of sonographer Christina Andrews to see babies in positions that their mothers can map once given a method for what they feel.
Bottom row: Dr. Bootstaylor and this mother bond over this experience. Her baby's back arm was down, just as she drew it. Everyone felt the magic of the evening!

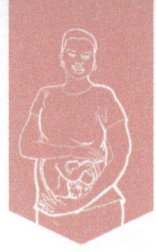

Cultivating Confidence
The Confidence Connection

Research demonstrates that strong prenatal attachment contributes to better child developmental outcomes, including enhanced cognitive, behavioral, and emotional development. When mothers develop a secure emotional bond with their babies during pregnancy, they're more likely to be sensitive and responsive caregivers after birth. This responsive caregiving style is crucial for developing what psychologists call "secure attachment," which is a fundamental building block of confidence and emotional resilience in children.

Children who experience secure attachment relationships typically display:
- Greater self-confidence and willingness to explore their environment
- Better emotional regulation and coping skills
- Stronger social relationships with peers
- Higher academic achievement and persistence in challenging tasks
- More positive self-concept and belief in their own abilities

Three Practices for Building Confidence

Based on the research findings, here are three practical techniques to strengthen your prenatal bond:

1. **Set intentions:** Find a quiet, comfortable space and place your hands on your belly. Take deep breaths and direct your attention entirely to your baby. Share your intentions with them about the kind of parent you plan to be and the hopes you have for them.
2. **Notice your baby's strength:** When you feel your baby's strong movements, you may want to push back gently and tell your baby, proudly, about the kind of power and strength they are already expressing.
3. **Remember your power:** Call to mind moments in your life when you felt powerful, capable, and confident. These moments will serve you as you think about the strong person that your baby comes from and the strong person that they are becoming.

A Lifelong Investment

The nine months of pregnancy represent a unique window of opportunity to begin building your child's confidence from the very beginning. Every moment you spend connecting with your baby, every conversation you have, and every feeling of love and protection you experience contribute to their future emotional strength and resilience.

Reference
McNamara, J., Townsend, M. L., & Herbert, J. S. (2019). A systemic review of maternal wellbeing and its relationship with maternal fetal attachment and early postpartum bonding. PLOS One, 14(7), e0220032. https://doi.org/10.1371/journal.pone.0220032

Step #3
Name Baby's Position

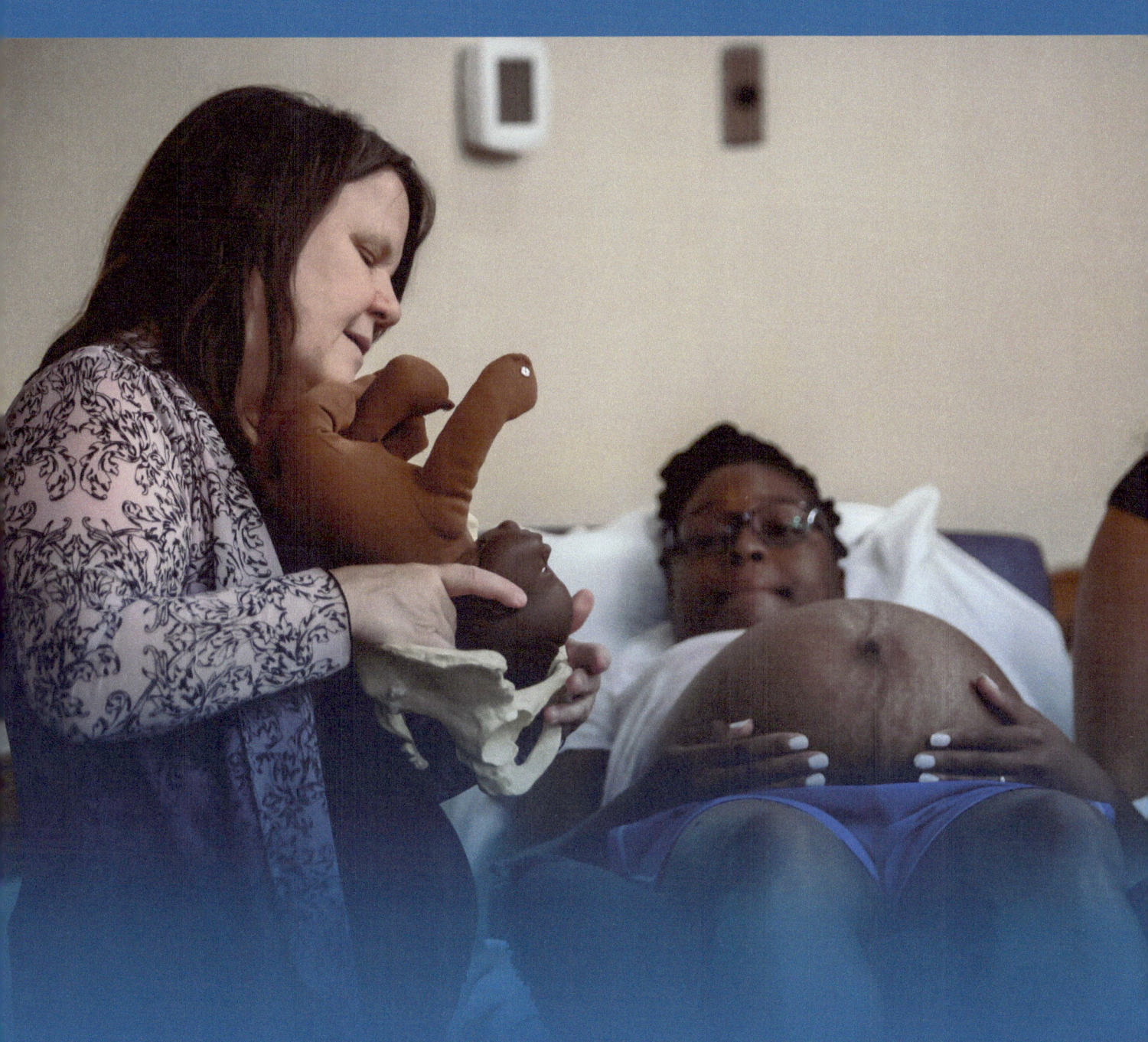

Step 3: Name Baby's Position

Now that you've mapped and visualized your baby's position, the final step in The Belly Mapping® Method is discovering the name of your baby's position.

It's OK to skip this step. This step may help, though, if you hear your doctor or midwife use fetal position names or you get curious and look up what to do at **SpinningBabies.com** or in our *How Baby's Position Affects Labor* section (page 69).

How to Name Your Baby's Position
The names for fetal positions are a bit like a code. All you have to do to crack the code is answer three questions. We'll help make the Latin words easy for you!

With what you know so far, answer three questions in this specific order. Choose the best answer for what you believe to be true. You can change later.

Question 1	**Where is your baby's back?**
Possible Answers	Left, right, anterior (front), or posterior (back)
Explanation	The back of baby's head is usually the same as baby's back. Pick where you feel most of your baby's back: on your left, right, anterior (front), or posterior (back). In birth talk, the words *anterior* and *posterior* are not used in answers for Question 1, so this answer is left blank. That's because these words are used later, among the

Let's go over each of the answers for Question 1 with sensation maps.

Left
You would have picked this answer if you feel the fullest and firmest part of the baby on your left and baby kicks on your right side. Hands might not be felt.

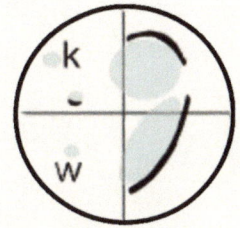 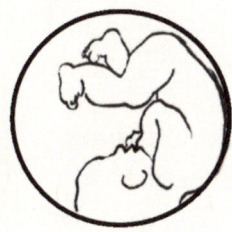

Right
You would have picked this answer if you feel the fullest and firmest part of the baby on your right and the kicks on your left side. You may or may not feel hands low by your bladder.

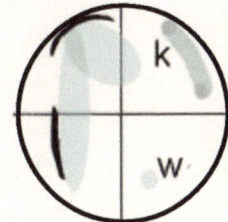 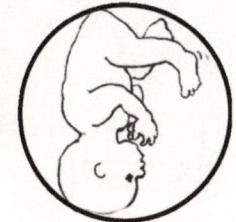

Back (Back-to-Back, Posterior)
You would have picked this answer if it's hard to be sure what I mean by "the fullest and firmest part of the baby." The back you may find isn't as big as in the other descriptions. You will see small parts in all four quadrants, but some areas will be busier or firmer than others. Knees slide by your navel sometimes.

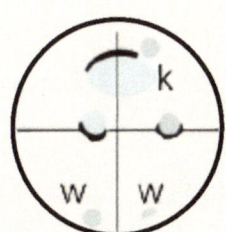 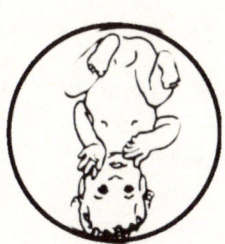

Front (Anterior)
You would have picked this answer if you feel the fullest and firmest part of the baby in front. The kicks are usually on the upper right, but for some, they may be on the left (unless limbs are hidden by an anterior placenta). The bulge slides left or right, but you don't feel hands wiggling, only feet kicking. Near term, the cervix twinges.

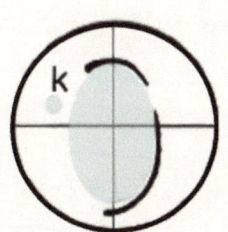 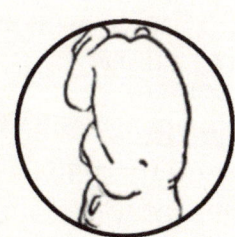

Question 2	**Which part of your baby comes into your pelvis first?**
Possible Answers	Occiput, *frontum*, *mentum*, or *sacrum*
Explanation	If your baby is head down, the presenting part is the occiput, the bone that shapes the back of the skull. In two rare head-down variations, babies present face-first with the mentum (Latin for "chin") or forehead-first with the frontum (Latin for "brow").

If your baby is breech, the buttocks, or sacrum at the bottom of the spine, are first. Some breech babies come out feet first, but sacrum is still the name used. |

Let's go over each of the answers for Question 2 on the presenting part.

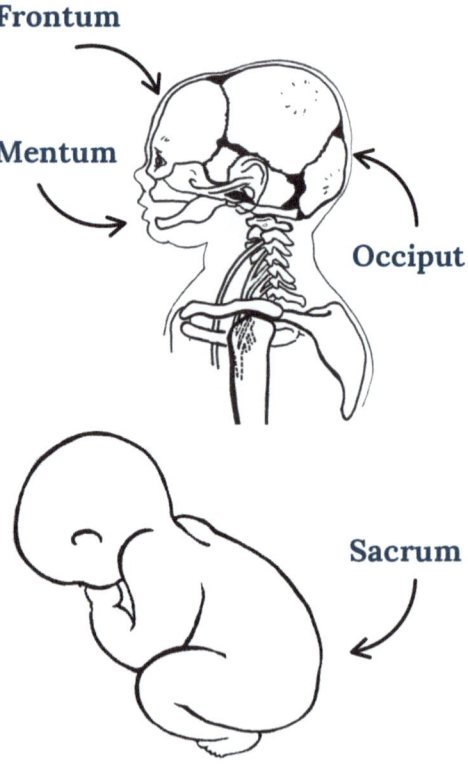

Occiput
The baby's **occiput** is the back of the head. The skull has several plates linked together with zigzag sutures (stabilizing without fusing). The "crown" includes this and two other bony plates.

Frontum
The forehead is coming first; brow presentation.

Mentum
When the baby's face is coming first; a face presentation. The chin is the landmark.

Sacrum
When baby is head up and coming buttocks or pelvis before the head (breech), the sacrum is the landmark we use. Feet, knee(s), or folded legs can come before the sacrum, but the sacrum is out before the head.

Question 3	**Which direction on your pelvis does the baby's presenting part aim?**
Possible Answers	Anterior (front), posterior (back), or transverse (head looks to the side)
Explanation	Your baby's presenting part may line up on your pelvis toward the front or anterior, the back or posterior, or back up toward a hip. We track the back of baby's head (or bum), not where the baby

Let's go over each of the possible answers for Question 3.

Anterior/Front
If you picked this answer, baby's back is along your abdominal wall. When you rub your tummy, you're rubbing baby's back, too! Feelings down low are twinges from uterine weight or the cervix ripening.

When baby is directly anterior, not left or right, skip the first word for the direction, or just say "anterior."

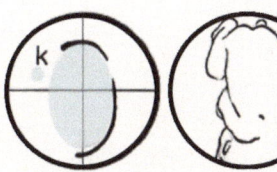

Left Occiput Anterior (LOA)

Posterior/Back
When baby is spine-to-spine, or sunny-side up, the face, hands, and feet aim to the front. Small knees slide beneath your navel.

When baby is directly posterior, not left or right, skip the first word for the direction, or just say "posterior."

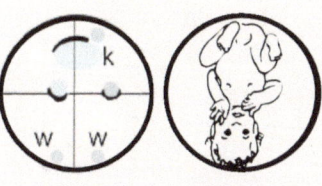

Occiput Posterior (OP)

Transverse/Head Looks to the Side
When a vertical baby is looking sideways in relation to the pelvis, the occiput (or sacrum) will be "transverse." You may occasionally feel a hand flutter on the other side of the center line from baby's back.

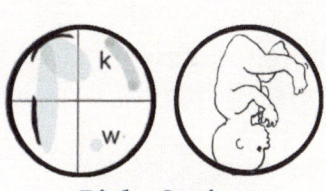

Right Occiput Transverse (ROT)

Fetal Position Names and You

Here's a visual aid for learning fetal position names.

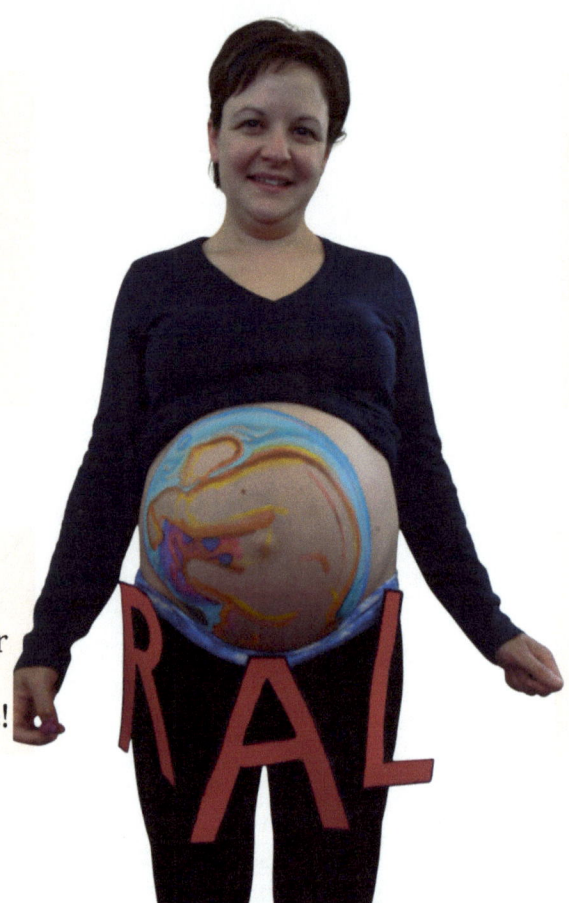

This side is our model's right side.

The baby's back is on this side when the baby's position name starts with the word *Right*.

This side is our model's left side.

The baby's back is on this side when the baby's position name starts with the word *Left*.

If an A, or the word *Anterior*, is the last word, it means your baby's back side is along the front side!

If a P, or the word *Posterior*, is the last word, it means your baby's back side is along the back side!

The letters worn by our model simply mean **R**ight, **A**nterior, and **L**eft.
Can you imagine the letter P on the back for **P**osterior?

Direction words in a baby's position name have to do with the pelvic bones. Where is the back of baby's head? The right, left, front, or back?

A for **A**nterior is along the front; baby is looking back.
P for **P**osterior is along the back; baby would be spine-to-spine looking forward.

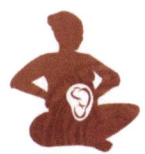

What is Your Baby's Position?

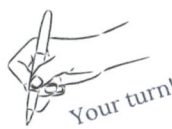
Your turn!

Write your answers to all three questions on the previous pages here. The three answers reveal your baby's position.

1._____ 2._____ 3._____

The first letter of each answer makes the abbreviation:____ ____ ____

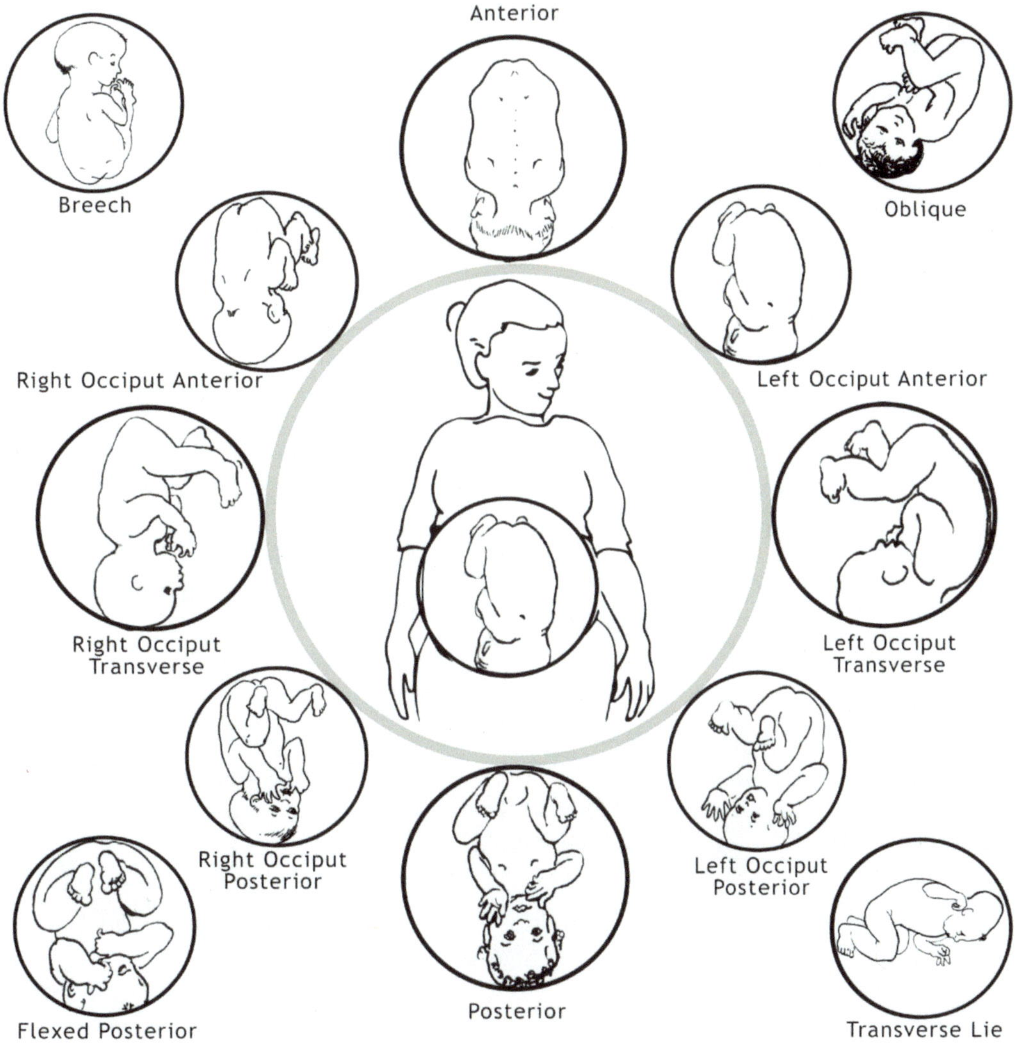

- Anterior
- Breech
- Oblique
- Right Occiput Anterior
- Left Occiput Anterior
- Right Occiput Transverse
- Left Occiput Transverse
- Flexed Posterior
- Right Occiput Posterior
- Posterior
- Left Occiput Posterior
- Transverse Lie

Is baby head up? See page 53 in The Belly Mapping® Method for a breech baby.

©2025 Maternity House Publishing, Inc. dba Spinning Babies®. All rights reserved. Spinning Babies® is protected by United States Trademark Nos. 4,200,336 and 5,527,742, and international trademark nos. 1,441,573 and 1,443,977. Spinning Babies® may not be used without permission from Maternity House Publishing, Inc.

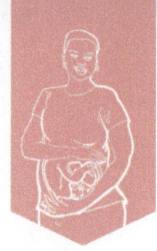

Opening to Love
Nurturing Baby Before Birth

The profound bond between you and your baby is deeply connected to the brain chemistry of love. The "love hormone," oxytocin, plays a vital role in forming attachment, empathy, and social behavior. By understanding how to encourage oxytocin, you can actively nurture your relationship with your baby in pregnancy, setting up a lifetime of healthy social connections.

Research shows that pregnant mothers with higher oxytocin levels tend to have greater empathy and stronger bonds with their babies. These oxytocin-rich prenatal experiences influence not only early bonding but also how we connect with others and behave socially throughout life.

The Lasting Impact of Early Love
What makes this research particularly fascinating is the understanding that early life experiences fundamentally shape our brain's capacity to produce oxytocin later in life.

When babies and children receive gentle, loving care, their brains learn to make more oxytocin, helping them feel safer, develop trust, form better relationships, and eventually become more caring parents themselves.

Three Practices to Build Oxytocin
1. **Gentle Touch:** Massage your belly with oil or lotion while talking or singing to your baby. Gentle touch boosts oxytocin and supports communication.
2. **Partner and Sibling Bonding:** Encourage partners and family to connect with the baby by placing their hands on your belly and breathing slowly together. These shared moments foster family bonding and help the baby recognize loving patterns.
3. **Mindful Movement and Nature:** Engage in mindful activities like walking in nature, swimming, or prenatal yoga. Being in nature reduces stress and promotes oxytocin, benefiting both you and your baby.

Building a Foundation for Life
Loving social activities naturally stimulate oxytocin production while developing patterns of attentive, responsive care. Gentle touch, warm connections, and loving care during pregnancy contribute to your child's lifelong capacity for empathy, trust, and healthy relationships.

Every moment of prenatal bonding is an investment in their future well-being.

Reference
Tarsha, M. S., & Narvaez, D. (2023). The evolved nest, oxytocin functioning, and prosocial development. *Frontiers in Psychology, 14*, 1113944. https://doi.org/10.3389/fpsyg.2023.1113944

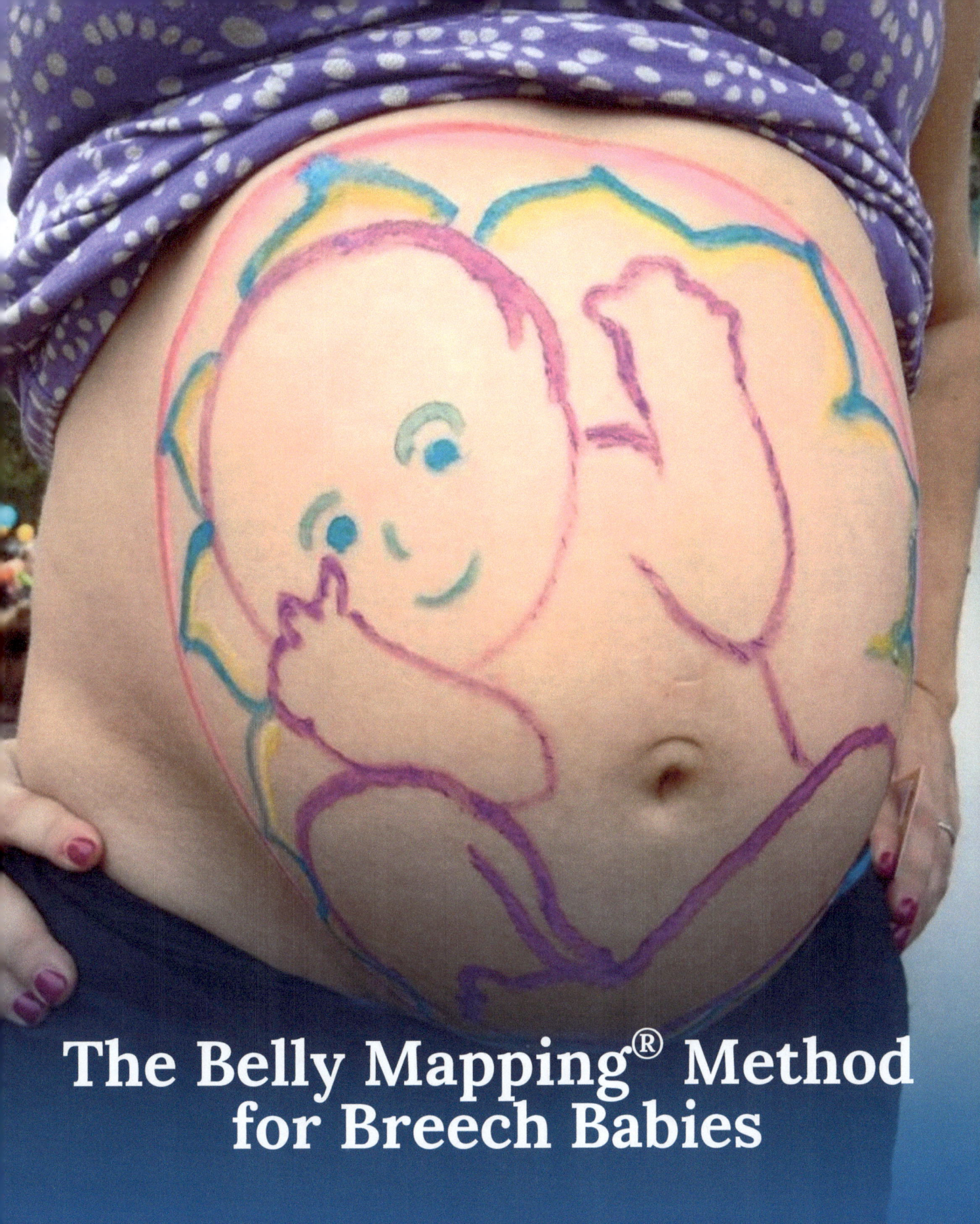

The Belly Mapping® Method for Breech Babies

The Belly Mapping® Method for Breech Babies

Most babies will settle head down by 30 weeks. By 32 weeks, 15 percent of babies are **breech**, and by term, 3 or 4 percent of babies remain breech. At the end of this section, there are some resources for you.

Every day, women and caregivers alike are surprised to find a baby in the breech position at the time of labor. Perhaps the baby flipped since the last prenatal exam, or the subtle differences between the hips and the head were missed.

Back in Step 1, we began to tell the head from baby's bum. Baby's head is near baby's back, but the bulge is not continuously smooth with the back. There's a short gap between the head and the back.

Here are tips to help you find out for yourself if your baby is breech or not.

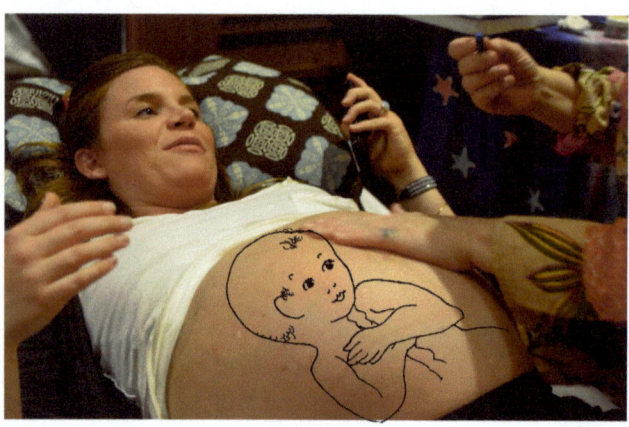

Naturally, we want to start with the head! Imagine a little baby with their head already snuggling close to your heart! Do you find the gap between the round head and the little shoulder?

Walk your fingers along the lower edge of the "ball." If there is no ball shape to the bulge, that's a clue. Keep counting the other clues.

Walk your fingers up the back until you find the little shoulder lump. There you'll notice a gap—your abdomen feels a bit softer right there, between the hard head and body. You've tried to find the neck from two different directions now. Remember to take a slow, deep breath to soften your abdomen.

- Feel the bulge at the top of your uterus. If breech, this will be the head.
- Find the gap between the roundish head and the broader back.
- There may be a hand near the head or gap. It will move independently and not "pivot" from the upper bulge. Check it over a variety of times to track it.
- Let your fingers follow the contours of baby's back. Can you find a shoulder?
- Is baby's bottom deep in the pelvis and out of reach, over by one hip? High?
- Can you feel legs or a single leg? It's unlikely you'll feel a leg if baby's legs are straight up along their torso. Read about breech positions on page 58.

The Belly Mapping® Method for a breech baby has a feel of revealing magic!

When a full-term breechling's back is to the front, the hips and head can feel quite the same. At that angle, the sacrum and head are the same width. When baby turns to the side, their sacrum feels more narrow and triangular. If the legs are straight and up by their tummy, it's hard to tell legs from the body.

You may be able to nod the head in the fundus freely without moving the trunk, whereas the trunk usually moves with the butt. Details can be lost behind strong abdominal muscles or a thick pad of fluff. The head may move over and back again over the course of the day.

Here are some questions to ask about what you feel:

- Does the bulge pressing out near the top of your womb make a spot on your abdomen warm or tender? That may be the head.
- Do you feel your breech baby "kick" near the top? Some breech babies' legs are straight along their chests and don't kick out. So what's kicking? Hands will move by the head and can be mistaken for legs, since there is no comparison.
- Do you feel a dip along baby's side? There is a dip at the neck between the shoulder and the head. Between the back and hips is a continuous firmness.
- Are the kicks or cylinders up top smaller than the kicks or cylinders near your pubic bone? Baby may be breech; arms are smaller than legs.

One clue might be misinterpreted, so it's more accurate to use multiple clues. If you aren't sure if baby is breech or not, compare two maps. Version A is for exploring a head-down possibility, and Version B for Breech, of course!

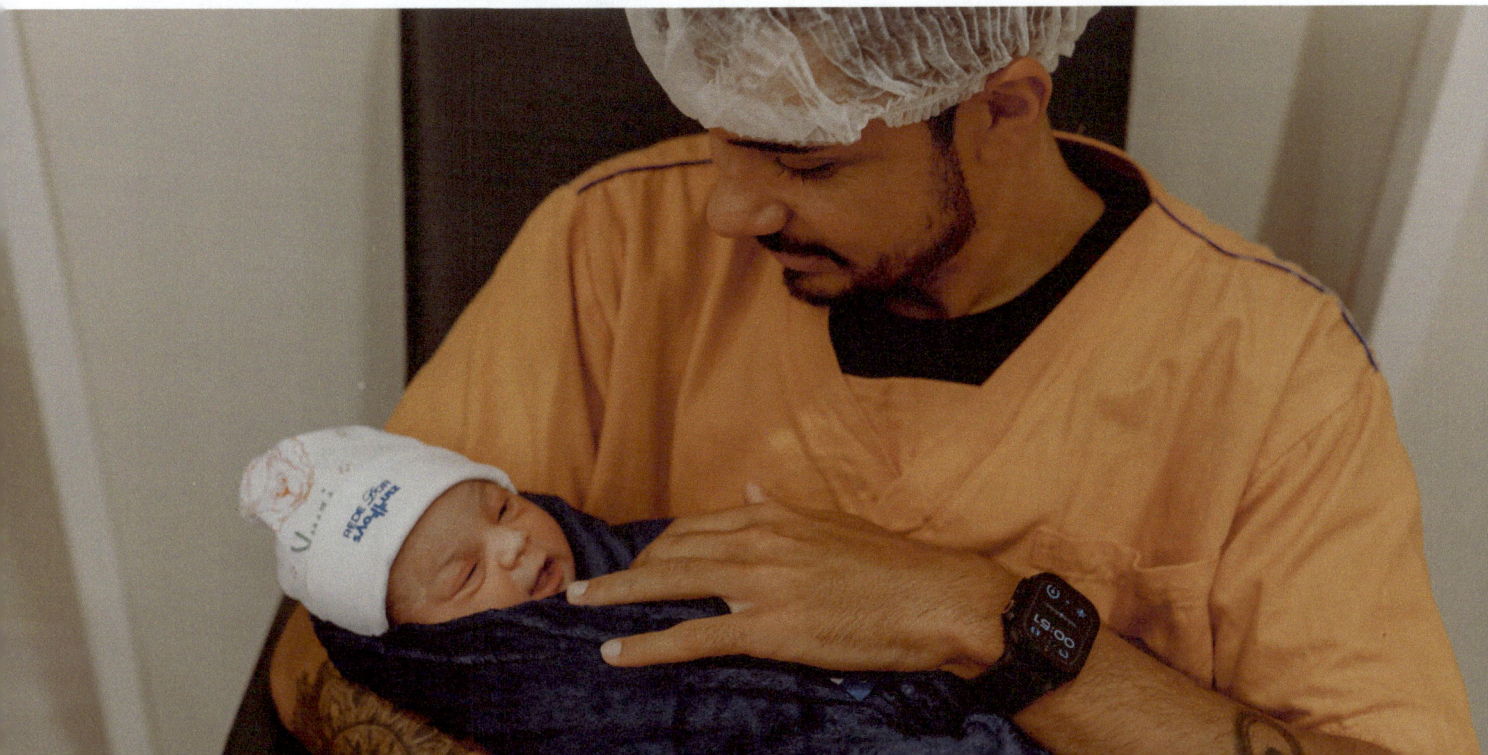

Bridget's Breech Belly Mapping® Experience

Hoping her breech baby would flip head down, Bridget was bold enough to feel into her situation. Literally. Reclining and relaxing, Bridget used her finger pads to feel her baby. She started at the top, exploring the contours of her son's head. Bridget felt her belly to discover which side her baby's back favors. Is it to the side, completely in front, or hiding in the back? On your map, mark your best guess or make a note in the margin if you can't find the back yet.

Next, Bridget checked for the buttocks. They may be deep inside, beneath the pubic bone, or sitting on top of the pubic bone, or they could be even higher. Not really sure where baby's butt was, Bridget found small parts the shape of cylinders near her pubic bone. Were these bent legs? A cylinder could be a thigh or a calf. She showed her guess by positioning her doll over her map.

Can you feel the little feet on your breechling? If not, it may be because of how the legs are arranged—for instance, if baby's back is in your front, the feet will be out of reach toward your back. Or the feet of a frank breech (see page 58) will be up along the body. Look first for the legs on the same side as the taps or small bumps (hands) at the top of your womb.

Being Compassionate with Breech
You, like many parents, may feel unsettled by sudden changes in the birth plan that arise when a baby is found to be breech.

Remember, there is no right or wrong to fetal position. Both you and your baby face a common human situation.

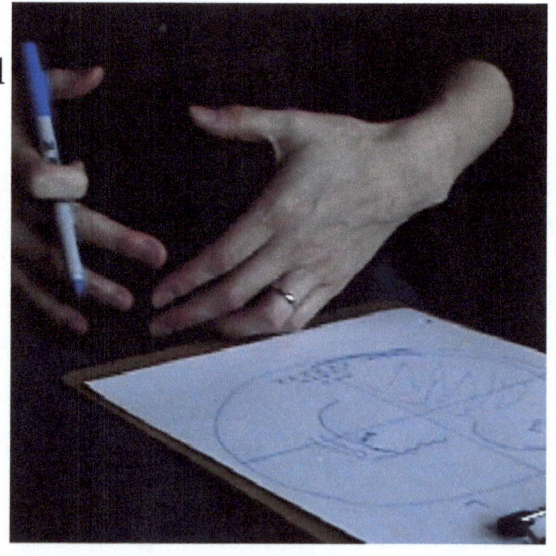

Being compassionate with yourself helps you navigate the unexpected, tune into new needs, and take steps to meet them.

Is there a match to your baby's position on The Breech Compass Rose? Page 81.

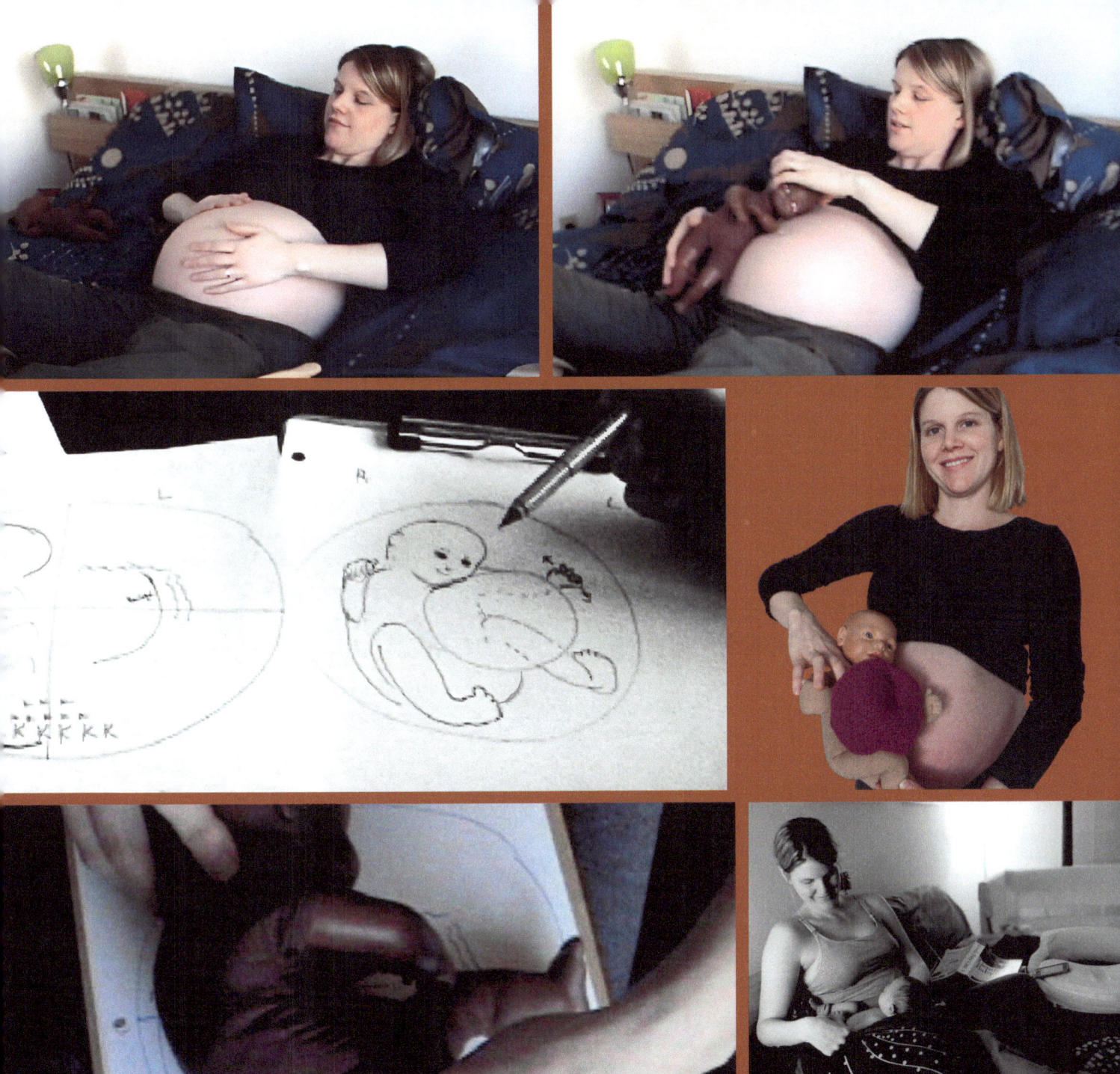

Bridget Tries The Belly Mapping® Method for Breech

Bridget realized her baby's limbs were behind an anterior placenta. In the above photos, she shows her baby's position using a doll and adds a knit hat to show the location of her anterior placenta. Bridget greeted her child by cesarean soon after these photos were taken.

Basic Breech Presentations

Frank: In the frank, or incomplete, breech, the baby's legs are straight up along the trunk. The baby's hips are born first. In a full-term baby, the hips and the head are the same diameter, so if the hips fit, the head will fit. A full-term, frank breech baby's legs are so close to the trunk that you may not be able to feel the legs by touch. You'll feel only hands on top, which means the "biggest kicks" won't be kicks at all!

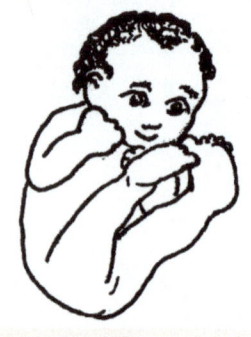

Frank / Incomplete

Complete: In a complete breech, the baby is positioned with the legs folded and feet to the center—something like a yogi sitting with knees bent. Thighs are flexed. You may feel the cylinders of the shins crossing above your pubic bone. Feet and knees shift near your bladder or slide by your pubic bone. You'll feel both hands and feet. Some complete breeches are called footlings incorrectly when their feet appear just lower than their buttocks. If the thighs are flexed near the baby's belly, and the knees are also bent, baby is a complete breech, even if the feet are seen first.

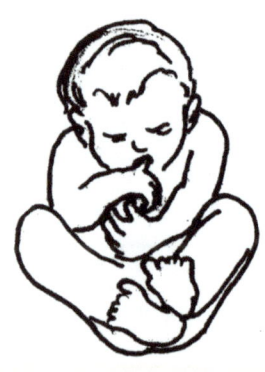

Complete

Footling: The footling breech comes with one or both feet first. Thighs are extended away from baby's abdomen; a footling's legs feel like cylinders leading away from the body. The bum is nearer to the navel than the pubic bone (at term). You may feel the feet "walking" on your cervix or bladder. A "single footling" has one leg up and one leg down. A premature baby is more likely to be in the footling position than a full-term baby.

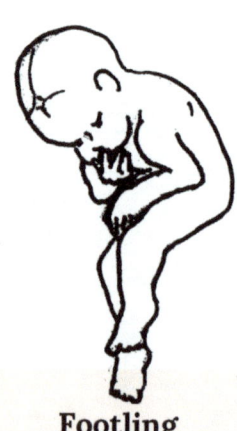

Footling

Kneeling: One or both knees appear before the buttocks or feet of the baby (not drawn here).

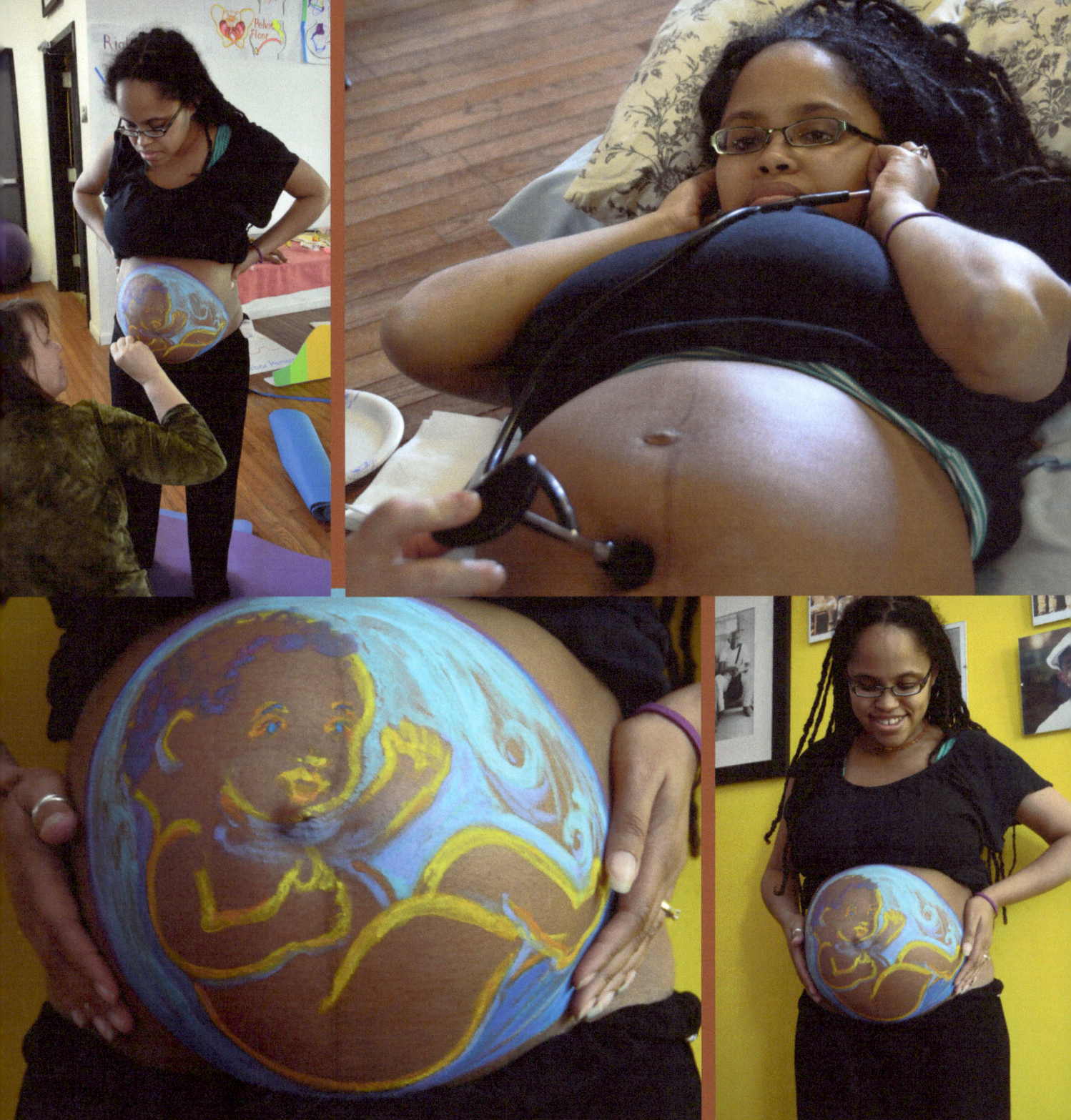

Breech Is Not Just a Position

Closeness with your baby reveals you as partners in your decision for how to give birth. The joy of bonding brings confidence that helps you explore decision-making.

Breech Position Sensations
Here are sensations for the breech babies who are posterior or on the right side.

Some sensations may be felt no matter which direction baby faces, depending on an anterior placenta or how the feet are positioned. Bent knees allow for the feet to kick more freely. Some breeches' feet tickle the cervix or kick the bladder.

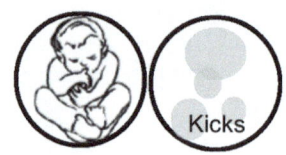

Sacrum Posterior (SP)
Baby's back is hard to locate. Baby's head may bulge in the top center. You'll feel baby's hands and perhaps feet all over the front, depending on whether the legs are bent and able to move freely or straight and unable to kick.

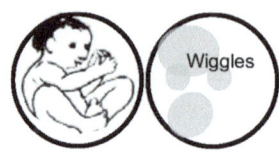

Right Sacrum Posterior (RSP)
Baby's back is only a little hard to locate, but you'll find it on your right side. Baby's head bulges in your upper right or top. You'll feel hands and feet over your front, but more to the left. You'll feel the hips aiming a bit left of center. Your care provider will hear baby's heart along your navel line, but far to the right of your navel.

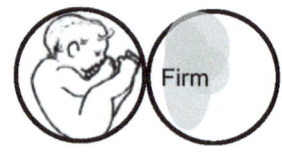

Right Sacrum Transverse (RST)
Baby's firm back is on your right. The womb is softer on your left. Baby's head bulges in your upper right. Sometimes this bulge is straight up in front, then moves right again, depending on whether there is room to move.

You may feel baby's hands and feet, and if you do, they'll be to the left of baby's head and back, but they may not be felt far to the left—perhaps more central. Feet may not be felt. Your care provider hears baby's heart on your lower right side.

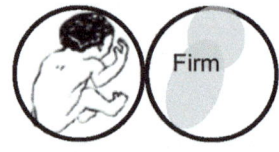

Right Sacrum Anterior (RSA)
Baby's back fills the front right, and you'll feel little parts only on your left, or on the left side of baby's head. You may or may not feel the feet move, depending on whether baby's legs are straight (the feet don't kick out) or baby's knees are bent (the feet have more room to move).
Your care provider hears the heartbeat easily on the front right, usually near your navel.

Baby's bottom may dip into the **pelvic brim** in engagement before the due date. You may feel cervical pressure from baby's hips being so low.

Here are sensations for the breech babies who are anterior or on the left side.

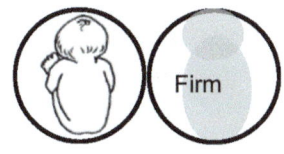

Sacrum Anterior (SA)
Baby's back feels firm in your center front. Arms wiggle on top and a little on the right. Baby's head presses up in the top center. Arms are towards the back. Your care provider hear's baby's heartbeat in a wide area in the front. Straight legs are not felt (or found by ultrasound), bent legs are.

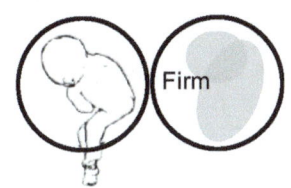

Left Sacrum Anterior (LSA)
Baby's back is on your front left. Arms wiggle on top and a little on the right. Baby's head presses up in your top left and occasionally in the center. You may or may not feel baby's feet, which are on the right. Your care provider can easily hear the heartbeat left and center, along your navel line.

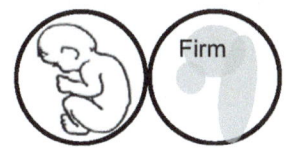

Left Sacrum Transverse (LST)
Baby's back is on your left side and may swing forward temporarily. Baby's head is in your upper left. The arms are clearly in your upper right and sometimes arc across the top of the womb as they move near or far from the head.

The legs and feet may kick or wiggle in your middle or lower right. You may or may not feel baby's feet. The lower half of your belly is quiet with a frank breech. Baby may feel low, causing pressure twinges on the cervix and upper thigh. Your care provider easily hears the heartbeat left and center.

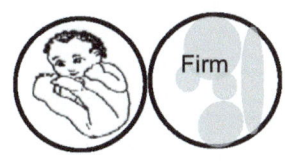

Left Sacrum Posterior (LSP)
Baby's back is on your left, but not close to the surface, so you may feel some softness on your left where you expect the back. Baby's head bulges in the upper left. Hands and feet move all over your front but favor your right.

Baby may shift from vertical to slightly diagonal. However, unless their bottoms are in a hip area, they are still in a breech lie. Baby may also swing their trunk from far to the side to more anterior or more posterior, but if the limbs are on the same side as before, an eighth of a turn in position isn't significant.

Activities for Flipping a Breech & Transverse Lie

Begin balance activities in midpregnancy to increase the likelihood of your baby being head down. Begin specific breech-flipping activities at 30 or 32 weeks for non-head-down babies. Make body balancing a daily priority! Continue regular balance activities to allow baby room to stay head down and/or ease the birth.

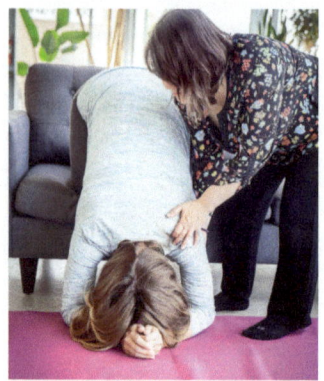
Forward-leaning Inversion

Forward-leaning Inversion (FLI)
This position is held for only 30-45 seconds for balance in pregnancy. Do this before the Breech Tilt or Open-knee Chest to make room for gravity to do its thing.

Get the safety warnings and specialized instructions to avoid turning your baby breech or harming yourself at SpinningBabies.com, or ask a Spinning Babies® Certified Parent Educator to teach you and a birth partner.

How does this work? The weight of the uterus stretches the cervical ligaments so that when you come up (carefully!), your uterus will align and make room for baby's head.

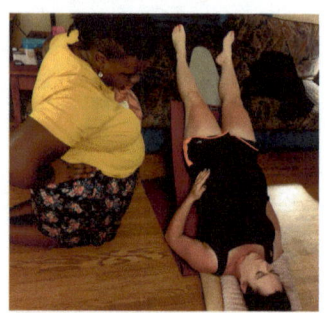
Breech Tilt

The Breech Tilt
This traditional pose helps breech babies settle their weight in your fundus to tuck the chin before a flip. It brings baby's bottom out of the pelvis. Repeat 2-3 times a day.

Use a firm surface, like a broad board. Tuck your feet into the crack in the couch for stability. Absolutely use a pillow to support your shoulders and protect your head from overextension. That's important! Repeat 3 times a day for 15-20 minutes until baby turns. Don't repeat when baby is head down. Then, walk!

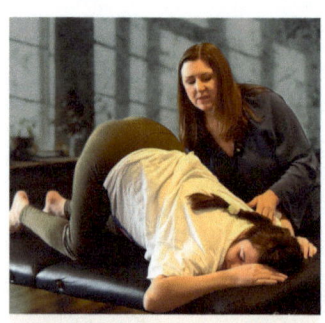
Open-knee Chest

Open-knee Chest (OKC)
This pose has also been proven to help more breechlings flip. Knees are only hip-width apart! Not wider! Just open enough to let your belly fit. Your knees are far from your belly, not straight under your hips. Your thighs and spine make a letter A that's "open."

We suggest doing the FLI (above) before doing the Breech Tilt or Open-knee Chest for better results.

Also: Some mothers say to do handstands in a pool!

Muscle and *fascia* hold balance best when released of chronic twists or resistance. Fascia and other bodywork therapies may help release tension in the membrane covering the pelvic bones and *pelvic floor* muscles. Some you can do yourself and with a breech-balancing partner; others require a professional.

If your baby isn't head down by 34 weeks, Dr. Carol Phillips, DC, recommends the *Webster technique* on both sides of the sacrum at each frequent chiropractic visit. Dr. Carol adds a symphysis pubis correction and sacral alignment, along with Forward-leaning Inversion and Side-lying Release.

What Is the Webster Maneuver for Breech in Pregnancy?
A chiropractor gets certified in the Webster Maneuver to release tension in the *round ligaments* and sacrum. Studies show a higher success rate in allowing a breech baby to turn on their own compared to "wait-and-see." Moxibustion, *acupuncture*, and hypnosis also have statistically valid success.

A manual *external cephalic version* **(ECV)** flips baby (a procedure with some risk) about half of the time. We recommend body balancing before and after an ECV to reduce force by first reducing the tension or torsion in the muscles or fascia.

Body Balancing Resources for Breech

Restorative Midwifery™ - Advanced self-care and "Breech Release" bodywork
- Breech for Pregnant Parents
  SpinningBabies.talentlms.com/catalog/info/id:143
- Breech for Practitioners Package
  SpinningBabies.com/product/breech-for-practitioners-package

Spinning Babies® - Simple home-centered care
- *Helping Your Breech Baby Turn*
  SpinningBabies.com/product/helping-your-breech-baby-turn-ebook
- Flip a Breech
  SpinningBabies.com/pregnancy-birth/baby-position/breech/flip-a-breech

General pregnancy-informed bodywork
- Spinning Babies® Aware Practitioners
  Spinningbabies.com/parents/spbap-directory

Dynamic Body Balancing® - Bodyworkers who've completed Dr. Carol Phillips's training, including craniosacral therapists, midwives, and chiropractors
- Practitioners **https://dynamicbodybalancing.com**

International Chiropractic Pediatric Assoc. (ICPA) **https://icpa4kids.com**

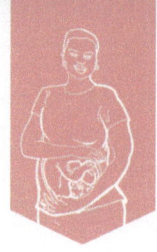

Communicating Kindness
Nurturing Baby Before Birth

Talking to your baby during pregnancy is one of the most powerful ways to begin a lifelong bond with your child. Recent scientific research reveals that prenatal communication shapes your baby's developing brain through the release of oxytocin. Understanding this remarkable process can transform how you think about those precious months of pregnancy.

Baby Hears Your Voice and Your Loved Ones, Too!

Your baby hears your voice as the second trimester begins. Along with internal sounds from your heartbeat and breathing, your baby hears outside voices and music. Babies have a remarkable ability for learning beyond sound recognition.

1. Your baby gets to know your voice really well. After birth, baby will feel calm and happy when they hear your familiar voice.
2. If you say the same words or sing the same songs many times, your baby becomes familiar with them. You may see them respond to these words or melodies after they're born. Babies won't get bored; they love repetition!
3. Babies can sense how you feel when you talk to them. If you're happy while talking, they connect those words with happy feelings.

The Chemistry of Love Through Words

Speaking lovingly releases oxytocin and dopamine in your brain—nature's bonding hormones. Regular oxytocin-rich conversations help your baby's brain start producing its own love hormones, supporting future healthy relationships, baby's nervous system development, and emotional security.

Three Practices for Prenatal Communication

Use baby's name or a loving nickname for them as you:
1. **Say hello:** Greet your baby in the morning, afternoon, and at bedtime.
2. **Read stories:** Read out loud while gently placing your hands on your belly.
3. **Sing songs:** Sing lullabies or your favorite songs.

The Lasting Impact of Prenatal Communication

Most importantly, don't worry about doing this perfectly. Simply being yourself and including your baby in your daily life with intention and love is enough. The most crucial ingredient isn't technique or perfect timing—it's the genuine love and kindness you bring to these sweet moments.

Reference

Petersson, M., & Uvnäs-Moberg, K. (2024). Interactions of oxytocin and dopamine—Effects on behavior in health and disease. *Biomedicines*, 12(11), 2440. https://doi.org/10.3390/biomedicines12112440

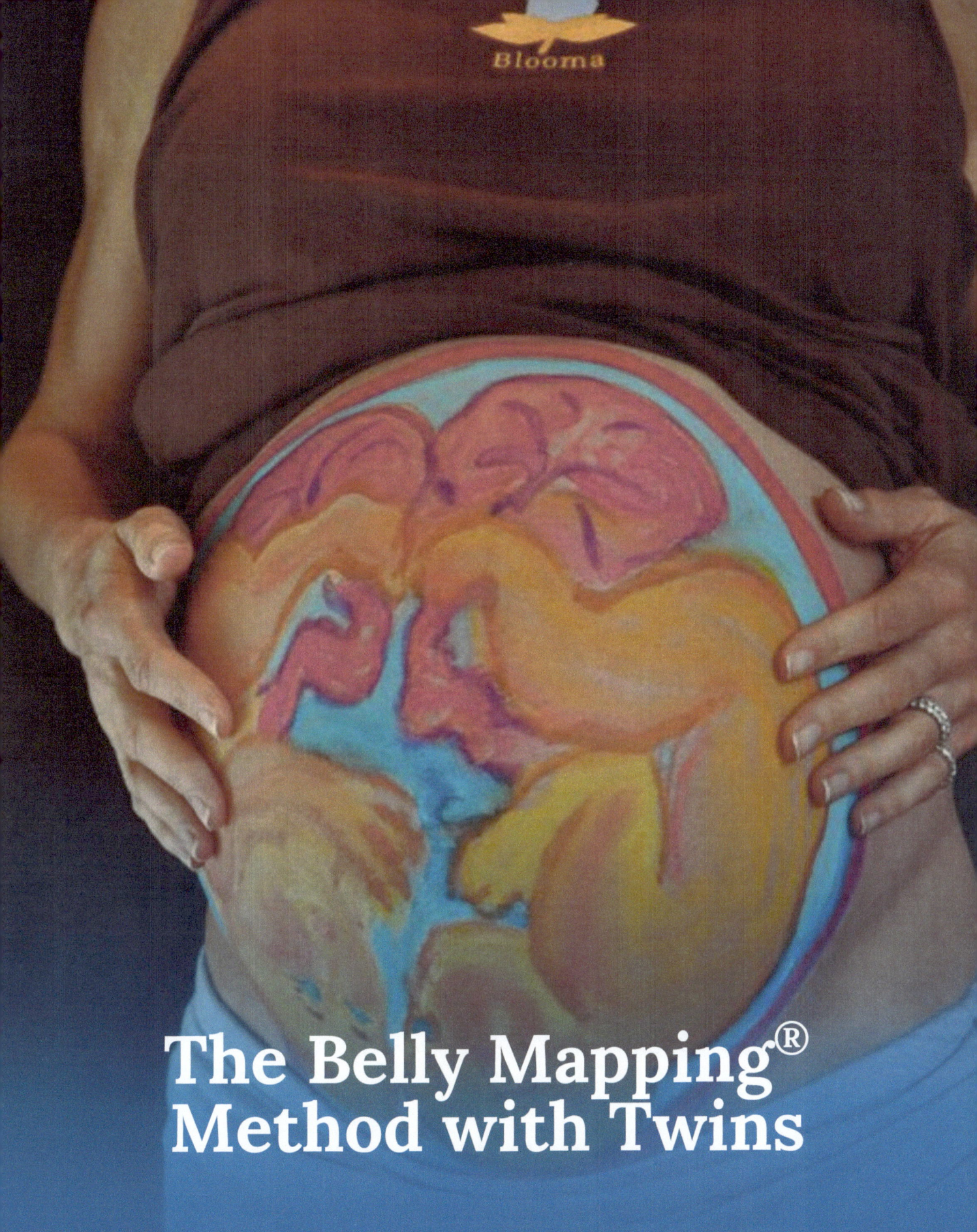

The Belly Mapping® Method with Twins

The Belly Mapping® Method with Twins

Two closely snuggled babies provide twice the bumps and wiggles as one.

Depending on how the babies lie, you may find two, three, or four big bulges. See if you can tell which bulge is a head and which is a bum by walking your fingers along one or both babies again and again. Pay attention to our clues, such as a gap between bulge and back (a neck?) or not (hips!). We can only estimate this way.

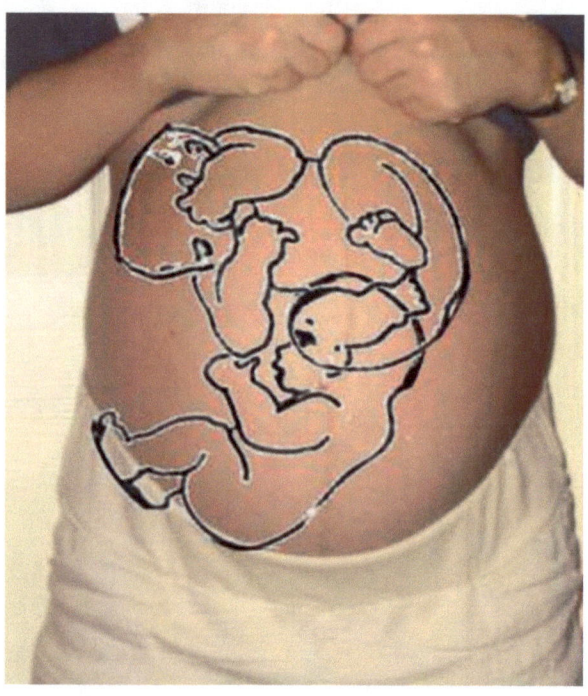

Telling Heads from "Tails" in Twins
1. First, find the biggest bulges.
2. Then, walk your fingers over each bulge and across any gap of a neck (or no gap) to find a smooth back or a front with less firmness and less smoothness.
3. Return to the same bulge and walk your fingers along the other side. Draw your findings on a map.
4. Feel deep just above your pubic bone to seek a head or bottom. Draw a circle on your map.
5. Find any cylinders: arms or the thigh if you feel it extending from a bulge (in that case, a bum). Draw what you are more sure of, and guess on the rest.

Twin positions influence options for vaginal or cesarean birth. Many care providers won't participate if only Baby A (the first twin in the pelvis) is breech, and some won't help you if both twins are breech (see page 53 for more about breech birth).

How often should ultrasounds be done? Reducing the number of routine scans may reduce the rate of lower birth weights from serial ultrasounds. Today, many twins are scanned throughout pregnancy, regardless of the evidence. The Belly Mapping® Method may offer clues about position change. Balance is for twins, too!

Debbie and Todd's Twins

Debbie planned a home birth in her pregnancy with twin girls.

Baby A was head down by 32 weeks. We weren't sure about Baby B.

Debbie wanted few or no ultrasounds, which was a common decision in that era and with home-birth parents.

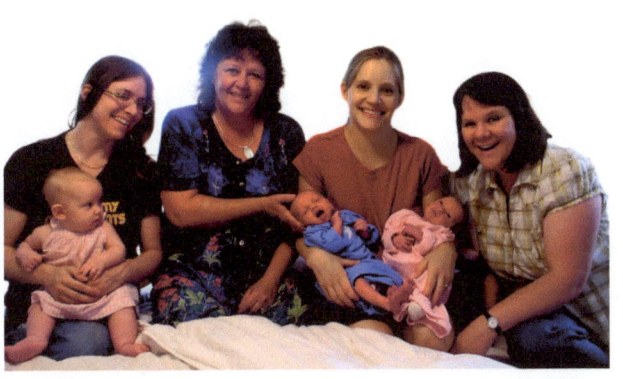

To help me visualize what I thought I was feeling, I drew two pictures (and laid them over photographs of Debbie's belly!).

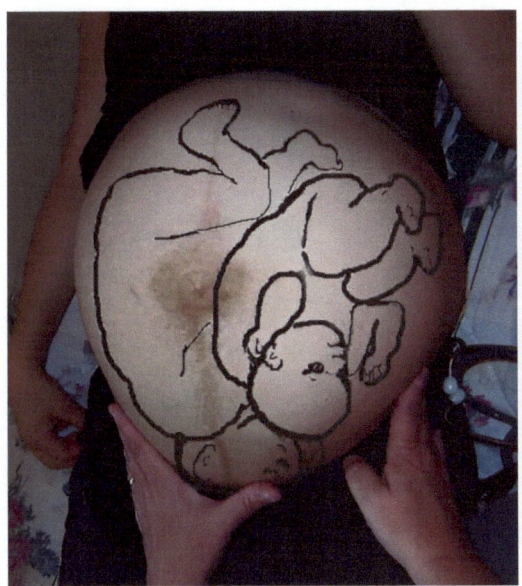 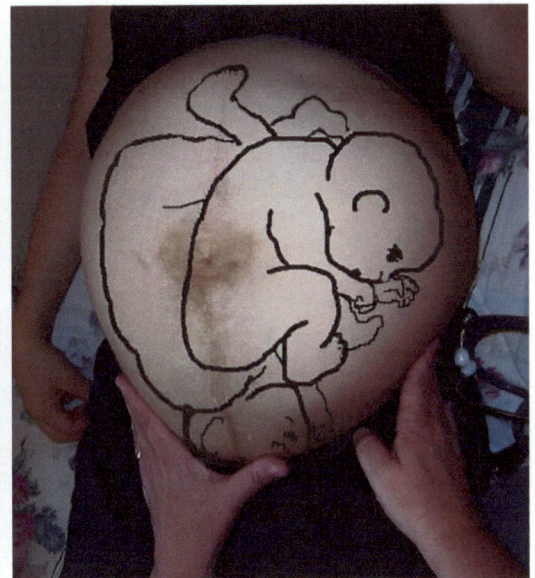

By switching the "poles" of Baby B., I could test which position made sense (left). Baby B was breech and was born full term and well.

Movements Become a Vital Clue

When you have so many bumps and bulges in your belly from two or three babies, the fun begins with figuring out which baby is the owner of which kick.

Older fetuses nap on a regular schedule—mostly while you're walking! So, see if you can identify which twin is which when one is napping and the other is moving. Then trace the moving twin's parts and begin to map just one twin at a time. The other twin will wake and give you a chance to follow their moves, too.

Step 2 with Twins
With these few hints, position your doll over your belly to match the bulges and the back. Adjust details as the babies reveal more of themselves over time.

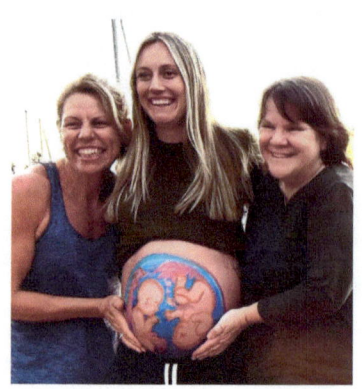

As one baby wakes, their legs may stretch to raise a bum and poke out a foot. This gives a clue to where that twin's legs are located. Sometimes you can trace a leg to the foot during this stretch.

Twins Interact!
If the twins are spooning or facing each other, you will feel both twins' bums and backs. Or you'll feel more of one's back. Or one twin is hidden entirely behind the other! Bring your map to discuss at your prenatal appointments.

Gretchen and Matt's Twins
Circles and lines on the left photo show bumps, bulges, and cylinder sensations for a breech Baby A and a head-down Baby B. Yet, an ultrasonographer reported the first baby was head down when labor began.

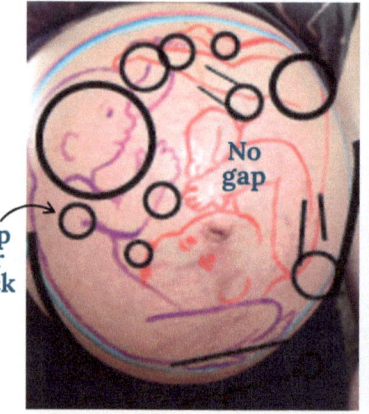 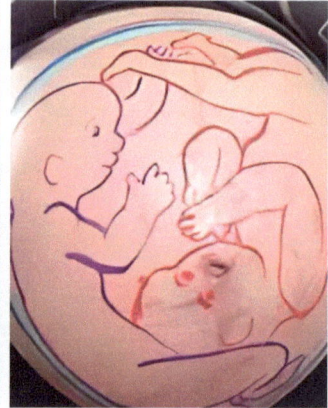

A sensation map is laid over the belly drawing of twins. Note lines show the location of limbs.

The Belly Mapping® Method must have been correct because two hours later, toes and bum appeared! Gretchen declined an offer for a cesarean and pushed out her breech/cephalic twins.

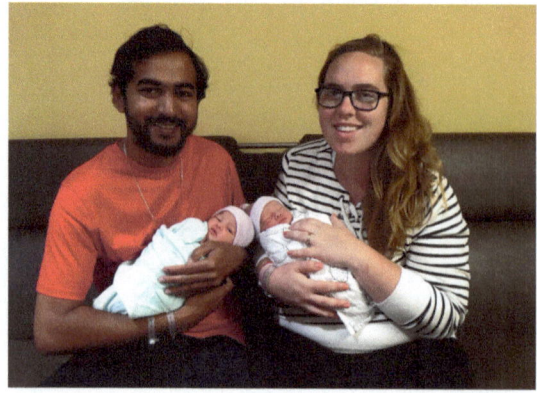

The Banerjee twins turned head down in labor with Spinning Babies®, just two hours before their planned cesarean.

Being Proactive About Twin Positioning
Encourage optimal twin fetal positioning through balancing activities in pregnancy.

Enjoy walking, breathwork, bodywork, yoga, and daily stretching. Ask your care provider if there is a medical reason not to do an inversion (such as high blood pressure) or our other recommendations. Help yourself reach full term with excellent nutrition, protein, greens, salt to taste, and cod liver oil (yep!), plus inviting and including more social support. Express gratitude now as if the twins were born on, or at, the due date.

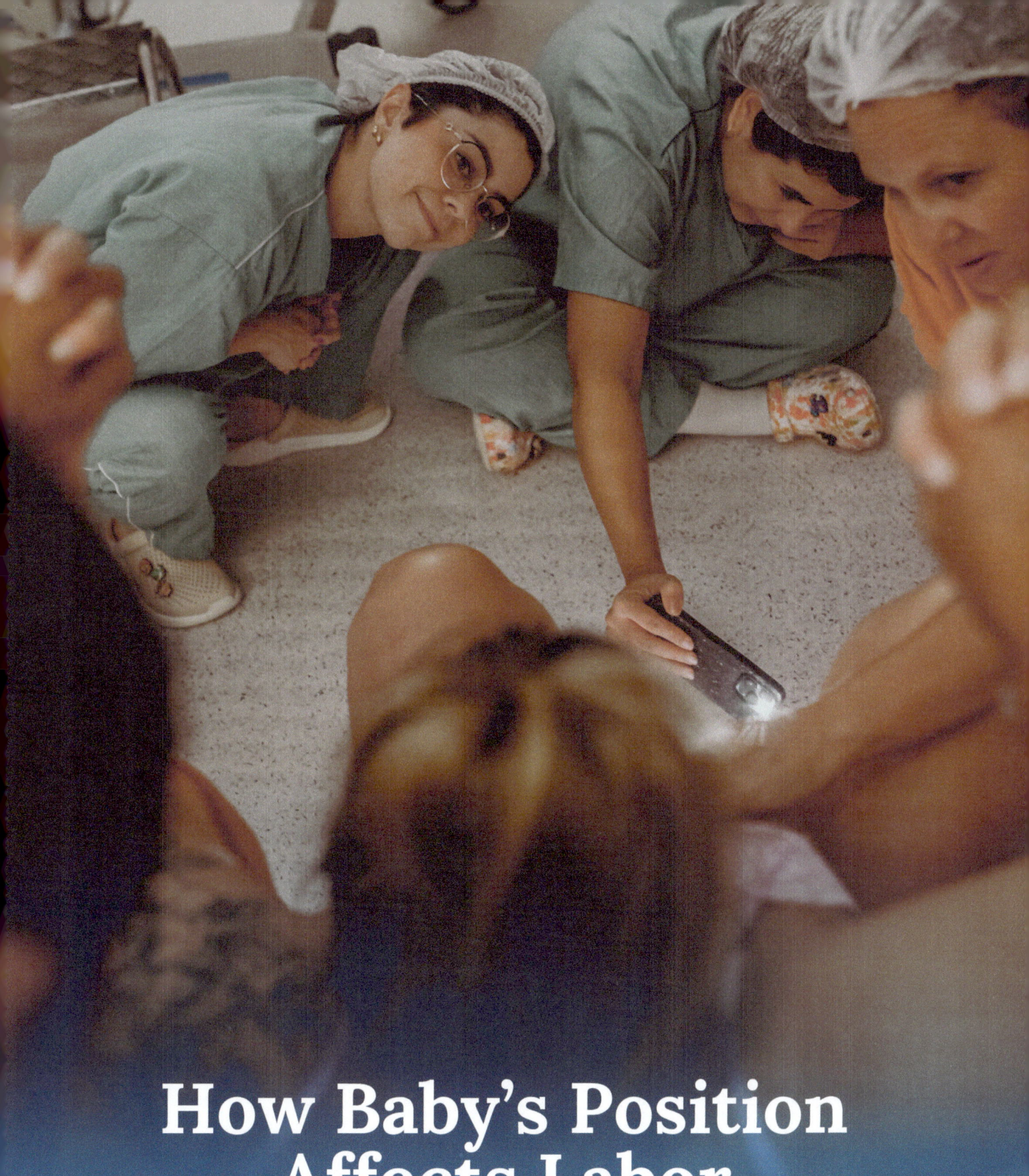

How Baby's Position Affects Labor

Baby's Position Fits on a Spectrum of Ease

Some fetal positions lead to shorter and easier labors, and some positions may more often lead to a physically demanding labor. For sanity's sake, however, try to understand that **baby's position** is one of many variables: an important one, yes, but not the only one. Those variables are in the next section.

May *all* baby positions inspire childbirth preparation! Keep *body balance as your superpower* in mind as you read this section. Body balance or imbalance is one of the variables that determine where you begin on the "**Spectrum of Ease**."

Spectrum of Ease

Spontaneous - Common Effort - Professional Help - Rescue

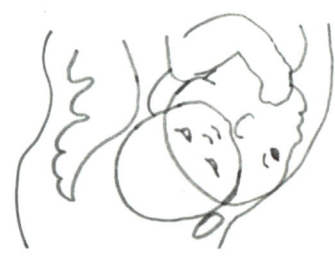

Here's one example: When baby's head faces forward, it may not fit, or it may be a tighter fit than if baby faces the right (back is on the left). Labor may need more help to progress.

As you look at the descriptions of baby's positions on the next pages, remember that adding balance will ease the path for any of the positions in which baby is vertical.

Add balance and then choose your birth positions to help baby move down the pelvis.

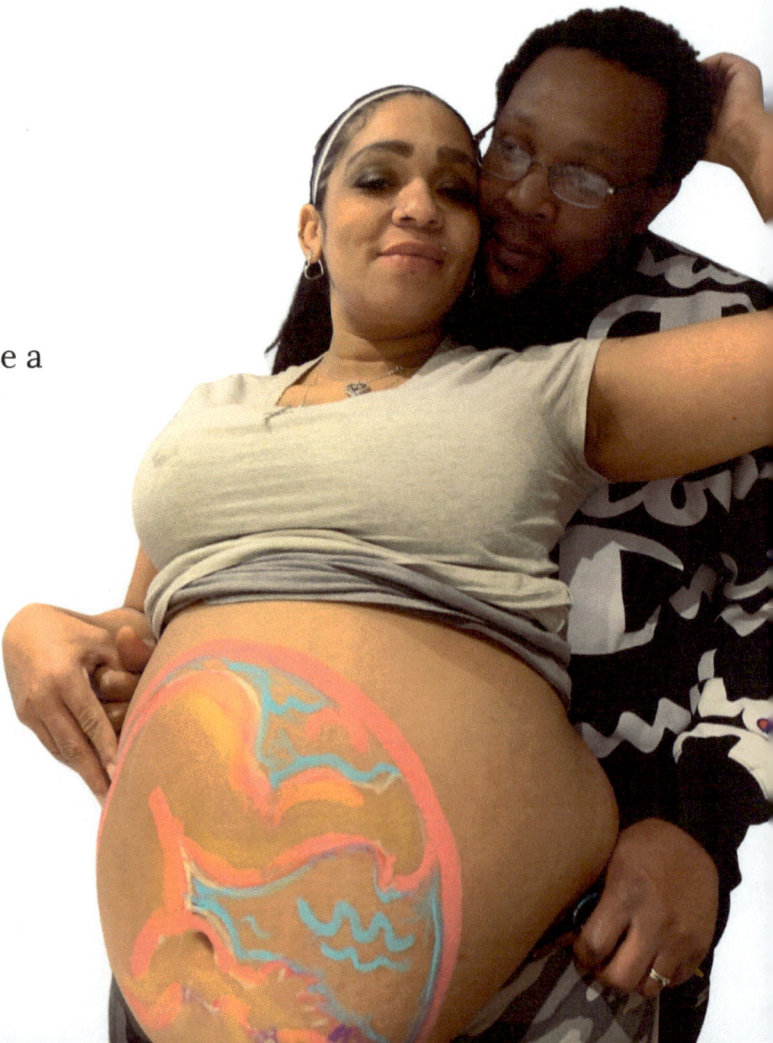

Baby Finds the Path in the Pelvis by Turning

Babies curl and tuck their chin to enter the pelvis. But which position do they turn to in order to do that? Turning through the pelvis is called **fetal rotation.** Baby turns to match the largest space at three places along the pelvic pathway.

In the literature collected over the centuries on childbirth, the **cardinal movements** of birth are those that *most* babies must do to fit.

The Cardinal Movements

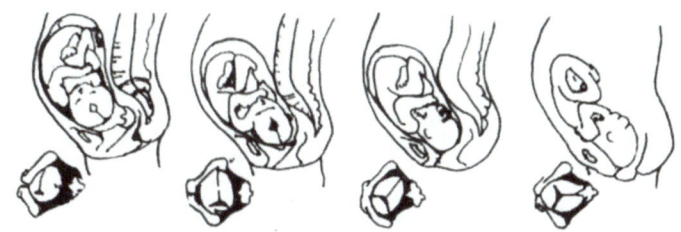

1. Engagement, 2. Descent, 3. Flexion, 4. Internal rotation

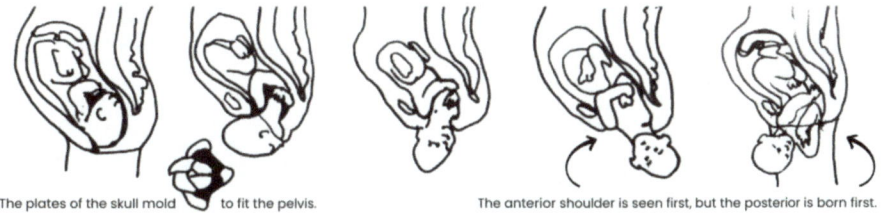

The plates of the skull mold to fit the pelvis.   The anterior shoulder is seen first, but the posterior is born first.

5. Extension (birth of head) 6. External rotation, 7. Expulsion

We see the baby flex their head and turn to fit each level: the inlet to enter, the middle or **midpelvis**, and the outlet to emerge. As baby's head is appearing, they arch their back to bring their shoulders into the pelvis. The chest and shoulders take the same turns to pass the midpelvis for the shoulders to emerge.

References

1. Holz, R. (2018). The 1939 Dickinson-Belskie birth series sculptures: The rise of modern visions of pregnancy, the roots of modern pro-life imagery, and Dr. Dickinson's religious case for abortion. *Journal of Social History*, 51(4), 980-1022. https://doi.org/10.1093/jsh/shx035
2. Hjartardóttir, H., Lund, S. H., Benediktsdóttir, S., Geirsson, R. T., & Eggebø, T. M. (2021). When does fetal head rotation occur in spontaneous labor at term: Results of an ultrasound-based longitudinal study in nulliparous women. *American Journal of Obstetrics and Gynecology*, 224(5), 514-e1. https://doi.org/10.1016/j.ajog.2020.10.054
3. Iversen, J. K., Kahrs, B. H., & Eggebø, T. M. (2021). There are 4, not 7, cardinal movements in labor. *American Journal of Obstetrics & Gynecology MFM*, 3(6), 100436. https://doi.org/10.1016/j.ajogmf.2021.100436

Engagement or Lightening: When Baby "Drops"
Engagement in early labor is common for women who have given birth before.

The first baby in a balanced body is likely to engage in the 39th week of pregnancy (and labor to begin on its own two weeks after engagement).

A first baby and those coming after a previous long labor or **cesarean** may need encouragement to engage to reduce the chance of a cesarean. Body balancing, active labor contractions, and certain birth positions will all help engagement.

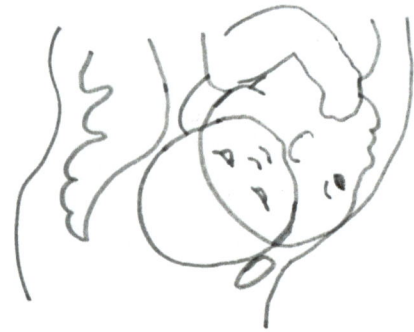

Baby turns to engage into the top of the pelvis.

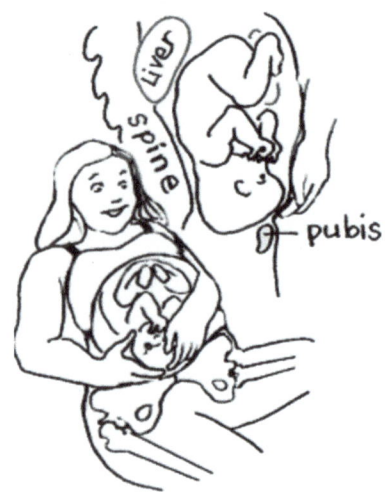

Is Baby's Head Overlapping the Pubic Bone?
Your baby's head is not engaged if it truly overlaps the pubic bone.

When you lie back, a head is overlapping when fingers feel a ledge or ridge made by the forehead as far out or even further than the pubic bone.

You may feel thumping or grinding on your pubic bone that occasionally hurts when the baby moves. (Compare this to loose pubic cartilage, which hurts when you yourself move.)

Checking for a Tucked Chin
Slide your finger pads up from your pubic bone. If smooth sliding, then press deeper to feel the sides of your baby's head.

- When you feel only one "corner" to the head, and it's on the same side of the baby as the limbs, this means the chin is tucked, or flexed.
- It's highly unusual to feel the corner on the same side as your baby's back. If you do feel one, though, then the corner is the occipital bone, or the back of the skull. This indicates your baby's chin is pointed up, or extended, which is associated with brow- and face-first babies.

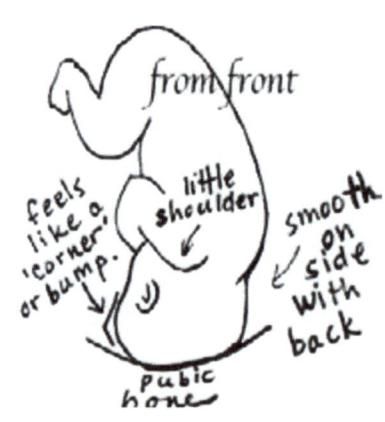

If the back of the head feels all one with the back, the chin is tucked.

Optimal Fetal Positions

The ideal fetal **starting positions** that begin an easier labor start with those that help baby tuck their chin, which happens naturally when baby's spine is curled.

Midwife Jean Sutton wrote the book on optimal fetal positioning. She was said to say Left Occiput Anterior (LOA) is the only optimal position. She did not.

Sutton made the point, and new research agrees, that short labors *more often* begin with baby on the left side than on the right side or spine-to-spine.

Babies on the left side are likely to be able to tuck their chins and aim the crown of the head into the pelvis, Sutton says. The round crown turns easier than the flat top of the head, allowing position change.

However, a few babies on the left can't tuck their chins. A few babies on the right can tuck their chins, making a vaginal birth more likely.

There are several variables in birth: fetal position, the bony pelvis, the pelvic muscle tone, health, whether premature or postdates, birth positions, size, hormones, birth skills in the team, and even the barometer dropping before a storm!

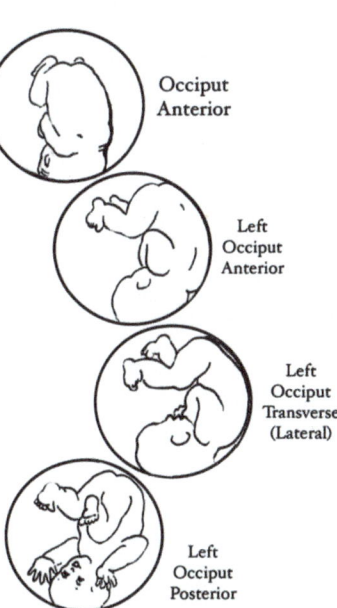

References Used Throughout This Section

1. Ahmad, A., et al. (2014). Association between fetal position at onset of labor and mode of delivery: a prospective cohort study. *Ultrasound in Obstetrics & Gynecology*, 43(2), 176-182.
2. Foggin, H. H., et al. (2022). Labor and delivery outcomes by delivery method in term deliveries in occiput posterior position: a population-based retrospective cohort study. *AJOG Global Reports*, 2(4), 100080.
3. Eide, B., et al. (2024). Associations between fetal position at delivery and duration of active phase of labor. *Acta Obstetricia et Gynecologica Scandinavica*, 103(9), 1888-1897.
4. Hjartardóttir, H., et al. (2021). When does fetal head rotation occur in spontaneous labor at term: results of an ultrasound-based longitudinal study in nulliparous women. *American Journal of Obstetrics and Gynecology*, 224(5), 514-e1.
5. Sutton, J., & Scott, P. (1994). Optimal foetal positioning. MIDIRS *Midwifery Digest*, 4(3), 283-286.
6. Tully, G. N. (2025). https://spinningbabies.com
7. Witkiewicz, M., et al. (2024, April). Perinatal Outcomes and Level of Labour Difficulty in Deliveries with Right and Left Foetal Position.... *Healthcare*, 12(8), 864.

Right Obliquity

About 70-80 percent of uteruses are higher on the right side. This is called **right obliquity**. Theories say the uterus has to shift to the right as it grows to fit next to the colon. Whatever the reason, this asymmetry is normal.

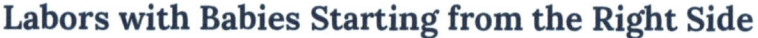

The result is that the right side of the uterus is flatter and steeper. The left side is rounder. Babies curl into the left and tuck the chin or back up into the right, lifting the chin.

In the literature, you sometimes see the term *obliquity of the uterus* to mean both normal right obliquity and also torsion of the pelvis, which is explained on page 16.

Labors with Babies Starting from the Right Side

Researcher Ahmad found 34.8 percent of fetuses started labor from the right side, while Witkiewicz found 81 of the 152 women in their study had babies on the right side; 71 were on the left. (Witkiewicz didn't look at direct OP or OA babies).

Labors with babies on the right side were longer. There was more **epidural** anesthesia given, and more labors needed a cesarean finish (11.3% vs. 37.5%, again not comparing front and back, but left and right). Vaginal births starting with babies on the right had more tears than those with the baby on the left.

Why Be More Proactive If Baby Is on the Right?

The reason is because when baby's back is flat against the steep right uterine wall, their lifted chin makes their head seem bigger. More importantly, though, is that baby's straight back means they can't use their spines to push and shift their head and shoulders lower down the pelvis like their friends with curled backs.

What Can You Do?

No surprise: **body balance**! If a person has pushed a baby out before, this labor has a good chance of finishing vaginally. Keep reading on for things you can do.

The next few pages go over each fetal position. After that, we share the general things you can do to help baby manage their way down the pelvic pathway.

References for Right Obliquity

1. Matthews, L., & Rankin, J. (2024). Muscle–the pelvic floor and the uterus. In J. Rankin (Ed.), *Physiology in Childbearing*. 5th ed., Elsevier, p. 297.
2. Berkeley, S. C., & Stern, D. M. (1941). *Pictorial midwifery: An atlas of midwifery for pupil midwives*. 4th ed, Baillière, Tindall and Cox.
3. Webster, J. C. (1893). The Occurrence and Significance of Rotation of the Uterus. *Transactions of the Edinburgh Obstetrical Society*, 18, 149.

Does Anterior or Posterior Position Matter?

The angle of baby's head is often why labor differs for anterior and posterior. There is a hidden reason, too: The muscles and fascia need balance!

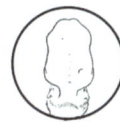

Occiput Anterior (OA)
7.6% of starting positions in Ahmad's study.

Starting labor in a direct OA position may have the following effects: The baby is most likely well curled, so the crown of the head enters the pelvis first. Engagement may occur shortly before labor or before labor gets active. Indeed, full engagement of the baby helps labor get active, and getting there will likely be smooth sailing unless there's some hidden stiffness or fear, not so typical with this position.

The labor pattern may be consistent, gradually getting stronger with contractions that get longer and closer together—the classic labor.

Suggestions
Upright positions may be effective on their own without a lot of snazzy body balancing. Comfort measures and calm companionship may be enough to cope. But be prepared with breathing styles and hot packs for active labor. Follow a physiological birth approach to finish vaginally.

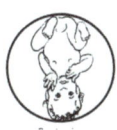

Occiput Posterior (OP)
4.4% of starting positions in the Ahmad study; Hjartardóttir found 52.5% at the start but 77% rotated to OA in labor. If the baby did not turn, 59% had cesareans.

The top of baby's head enters the pelvis first. The baby's back is arched spine-to-spine. Baby can't help from this position, so the birthing person is doing all the work while their little birth partner inside waits for every centimeter of space to scooch down the pelvis.

The posterior labor pattern can vary, but few are predictable. There's the "start and stop" pattern that keeps everyone wondering. Labor seems to start and then stops for hours or days. Or after starting, labor stalls out. Contractions can double-peak, or cluster, then go into a lull.

A posterior labor can be faster, harder, and more painful at 2 cm than at 8 cm. Sometimes the pushing urge is strong at 5 or 8 cm instead of 10. Most OP babies do turn at some point in labor.

Suggestions
Begin with body balancing in pregnancy—for the whole body. Activate the fascia with Side-lying Release for function and room for baby to turn or descend. Don't delay. Balance again in labor before the water releases or labor advances. Don't break the water; try an FLI instead! Be upright (and out of the pool) with birth positions that open the top.

Possible Effects & Suggestions for the Left Side

A left-sided labor pattern starts gradually, and though some contractions may take a leap forward in strength, labor progression is predictable. If you like, you can adjust your focus and breathing to cope. This labor has plenty of oxytocin!

Once 8 cm arrives, you'll likely need to upgrade your coping techniques to accommodate the release of adrenaline. Once 10 cm dilated, you may have a pause. Rest if you can. Let the urge build before pushing actively and then pant.

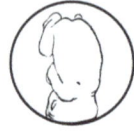

Left Occiput Anterior (LOA)
12.4% of starting positions for births in Ahmad's study. Witkiewicz found 13.6%. Baby's back curls up across the front. The head looks diagonally. This position is unusual to start labor because it will occur when entering a triangular-shaped brim in the pelvis, which is less common. A large baby can then be a special challenge, but the LOA labor will reward movement and effort. Birth position is sometimes critical.

Suggestions
Baby has little rotation to do, so that's not an issue. Open the bones! To let babies in the pelvis, do a **posterior** *pelvic tilt* with a contraction.

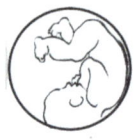

Left Occiput Transverse (LOT)
27.4% of starting positions in the Ahmad study; 15.5% in the Hjartardóttir study. Baby is on the left, facing the right. The most common position of the four flexed positions. Baby readily engages in, or enters, the pelvis before labor or in early labor.

A first baby in this position usually stays in this position until about 7 cm, when they will turn to Left Occiput Anterior until pushing, when they then turn to a direct Occiput Anterior position for birth.

Suggestions
Babies need added help if they *stay* in this position past 5 cm. *Side-lying Release* and side lunges or asymmetrical positions (***exaggerated lateral decumbent***, which is leaning over from the side-lying position).

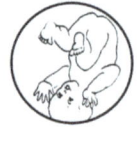

Left Occiput Posterior (LOP)
13.4% of all starting positions in Ahmad's study; 2.5% in Witkiewicz's study. The LOP baby may have a tucked chin to help rotate with little or no help. The tucked chin aims the round crown into the pelvis for easier turning. In thirty years of birth, I saw only three cesareans for LOP.

Suggestions
Balance and check the forehead: *Abdominal Lift and Tuck* to engage or to help a forehead come off the pubic bone.

Possible Effects & Suggestions for the Right Side

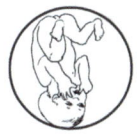

Right Occiput Posterior (ROP)
45.1% of babies coming down from the right side were ROP in Witkiewicz's study. Baby is on your right, facing out diagonally a bit to the left. The thing to check with this position is whether baby's forehead is resting on your pubic bone or tucked politely behind it. Getting past the pubic bone is necessary to enter the pelvis. The first goal, however, isn't engagement but rather rotation.

With usual care, moving freely, eating, and being upright, this position can take a couple of days or more to enter and move through the pelvis. The chance of a cesarean can be "turned around" if baby can turn.

The head position is a challenge, but the issue is not the baby; it's the chronic tension on the right side in muscles and fascia, which can be released, sometimes quite quickly, with a *Side-lying Release (SLR)*.

The Next Position After ROP
Baby may turn to a direct Occiput Posterior and then may engage. Or baby may turn to Right Occiput Transverse under the pressure of strong contractions. They'll keep turning to Right Occiput Anterior in a few cases, and some will swing all the way over to Left Occiput Transverse, and then the uterus will rest. When labor resumes, the labor will be easier and more straightforward.

Suggestions
If the forehead is on top of the bone, lift your belly during the whole contraction and tilt (flatten) your lower back (*Abdominal Lift and Tuck*). Help baby rotate to the front or left before engagement.

Baby's back is far from your abdomen, so the nurse or midwife often hunts around for the heartbeat with the listening device. When you or baby move, they have to hunt again. This is just because baby's heart is not close to your skin. Help baby rotate with an *SLR*, page 88.

Try not to force baby to engage by doing brim-opening positions before doing *body balancing* for the soft tissues that would guide baby into flexion if they had their tension released. Body balancing may help baby rotate to the left side before dropping into the pelvis.

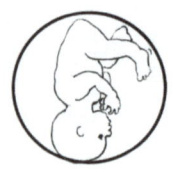

Right Occiput Transverse (ROT)
35.4% of babies on the right were ROT in Witkiewicz's study.
The baby faces your left hip. Whether baby rotates to OA or to OP depends on flexion and space in the bones. ROT often turns to posterior. Very strong contractions may take a day or two to turn baby to OP or ROA. If baby is able to turn all the way to LOT, labor takes a rest and resumes well. Easier than ROP (usually) and statistically unlike LOT.

Suggestions
Body balancing and care in birth positions may allow the baby to flex and turn to the left before entering the pelvis. Then labor will likely progress after a pause in labor (commonly).

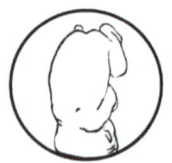

Right Occiput Anterior (ROA)
Only 3.8% of *starting* positions were ROA in the Ahmad study.
Baby's back is straight up on the front right side. The head is in a diagonal. This position is not a likely starting position but is often diagnosed (incorrectly). ROA comes after some posterior babies rotate as far forward as they can. ROA is more able to engage in the pelvis than ROP. ROA is often the birth position we see after an ROP or ROT baby turns to fit the outlet.

Baby's chin may tuck enough when in this starting position. Labor often starts with a normal progress pattern. The size and flexibility of the midpelvis can affect the length of labor.

This position is not a mirror image of Left Occiput Anterior, despite my drawing. The back is straighter; the chin may be up. Most ROA births can finish vaginally.

Suggestions
The mother's muscles may have tension that holds the baby high. Warm up the two **psoas** muscles draping over the front sides of the pelvis with forward lunges and even Walcher's position.

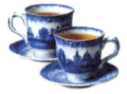

Uterine contractions help turn baby. Help turning becomes easier with stretches in positions that bring body balance. Labor is actually your body opening and releasing baby.

Possible Effects & Suggestions for Breech

There are few studies on the course of physiological labor for breech. These comments are based on my own observations and those of the people noted.

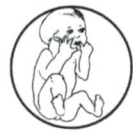
Right Sacral Posterior (RSP)
Baby's back is on the right, and the hips are aiming right into the pelvis. Labor may begin quickly and easily bring the hips into the pelvis. The pelvic floor turns the hips like a button through a button hole so the baby comes out the **pelvic outlet** from the left side. This is a favorable position for vaginal breech birth (VBB). However, whether cesarean or vaginal, a skilled breech provider reduces harm.

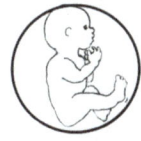
Right Sacral Transverse (RST)
This is a favorable starting position for a breech birth. Baby starts this way but may turn to Right Sacrum Anterior to fully engage. They will then turn to oblique and come into the outlet from the left (Evans).

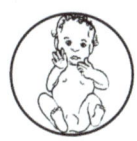
Sacral Posterior (SP)
This is a rare starting position and a rare ending position for a breech birth. However, this is not a safe finishing position, and the midwife or doctor would manually rotate baby to anterior to increase safety.

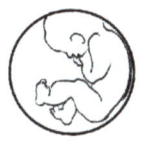
Left Sacral Transverse (LST)
While there isn't much research on how breech babies rotate, Jane Evans and Mary Cronk, UK midwife partners, noted left-sided breeches took longer, had to rotate further, and therefore were more often caught on the pelvis. Long latent phases occur, which can risk infection or become tiring, and a cesarean becomes more attractive or necessary. Midwife Diane Goslin waits it out with parents and finds most of these labors end vaginally. Extreme skill is needed here.

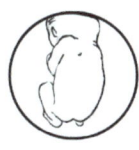
Left Sacral Anterior (LSA)
Similar to LST, the LSA baby finds the rounder left side of the uterus can aim them toward the hip more than into the pelvis. Balance and birth positions help avoid hours of waiting for contractions to engage baby's bum. Abdominal Lift and Tuck is a favorite of Nicole Morales.

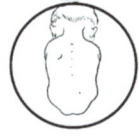
Sacral Anterior (SA)
As baby engages into the pelvis, they may take a sacrum anterior position. They will then do a small rotation in the pelvic floor to oblique and be turned back to SA for the outlet, theoretically.

Reference

1. Evans, J. (2012). The final piece of the breech birth jigsaw?. Essentially Midirs, 3(3), 46-49.

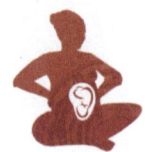

The Fetal Compass Rose
by Midwife Gail Tully

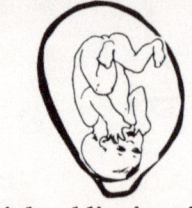

Right obliquity of the womb makes the right side steep and the left side rounder.

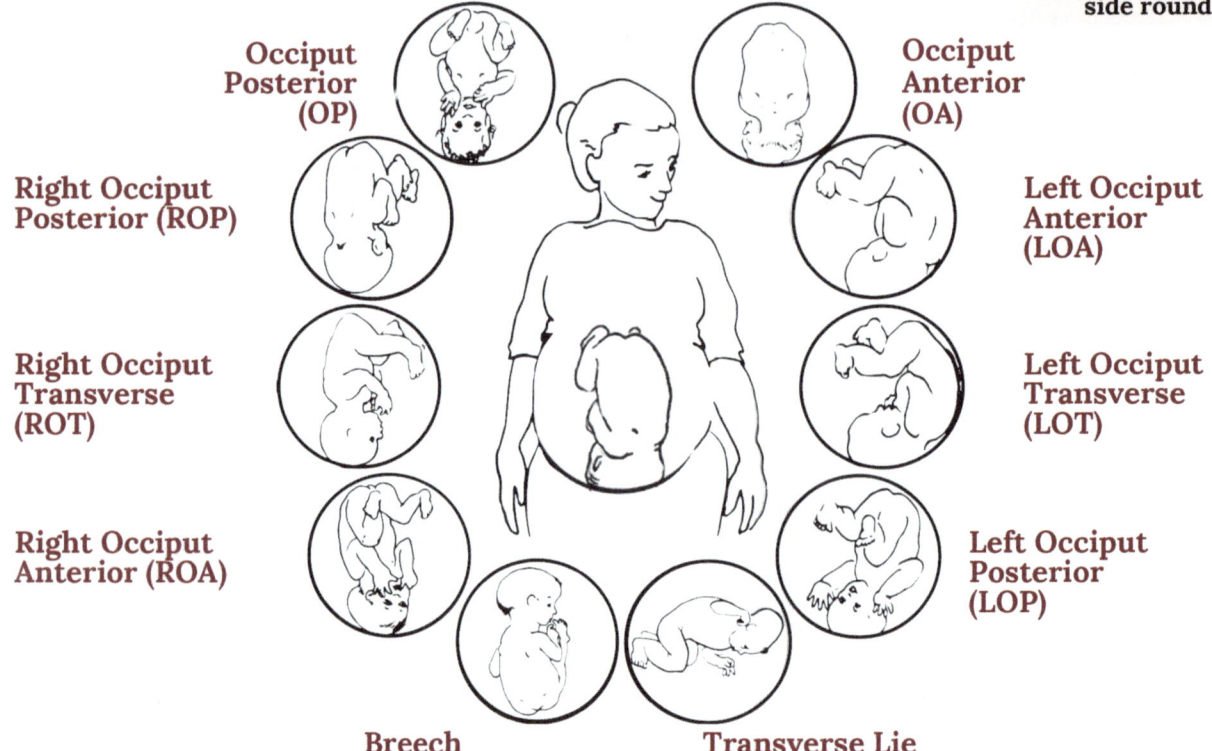

Breech Lie

Baby is breech when the hips will be born first. Cesarean surgery is often recommended. There can be several reasons why a baby is breech.

Transverse Lie

A baby lying sideways is in a transverse lie. Normal in early pregnancy, but baby cannot be born like this. SpinningBabies.com has a solution.

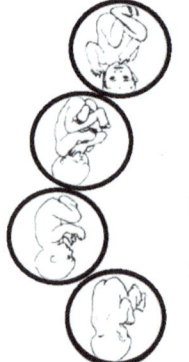

Posterior and ROA

Right obliquity of the uterus makes the right side of the uterus steeper. That straightens the spine of the baby on the right side and lifts baby's chin, aiming the top of baby's head into the pelvis. This lack of flexion may delay engagement, slow descent, and make pushing longer. Specific techniques to help baby rotate avoid a cesarean.

Anterior and LOP

When a baby's back comes down from the left side, baby's back curls against the rounder side of the uterus. Curling the spine will tuck the chin, which aims the crown into the pelvis so they can turn and descend well during labor. Labor contractions proceed in a dependable rhythm. A tucked chin allows head molding for easier pushing.

©2025 Maternity House Publishing, Inc. dba Spinning Babies®. All rights reserved. Spinning Babies® is protected by United States Trademark Nos. 4,200,336 and 5,527,742, and international trademark nos. 1,441,573 and 1,443,977. Spinning Babies® may not be used without permission from Maternity House Publishing, Inc.

The Breech Compass Rose
by Midwife Gail Tully

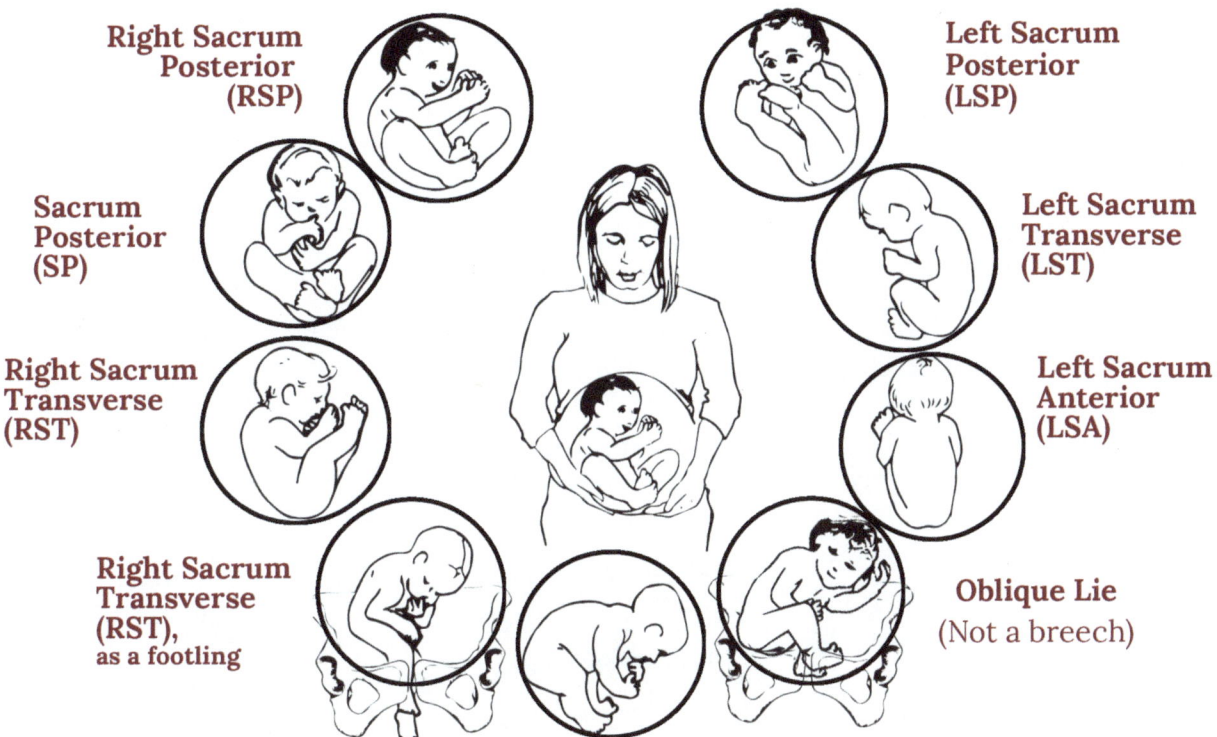

A Posterior Breech
The Sacrum Posterior baby looks forward. The pelvic floor turns most babies in this start position to ST; a care provider needs to turn any still posterior near the end, before the arms are out.

Transverse or Oblique Lie
A baby lying sideways is in a transverse lie. A baby in the diagonal is oblique. Normal in early pregnancy, not in late pregnancy. These are sometimes mistakenly called breech.

Right-Sided Breechlings
Right obliquity of the uterus makes the right side of the uterus steeper. That straightens the spine of the baby on the right side, which is helpful for a breech baby. Labor is more likely to be fast with fewer stuck breeches. However, any breech baby can get stuck, so have a very well-trained breech provider for a planned vaginal breech birth.

Left-Sided Breechlings
When a baby's back comes down from the left side, baby's back curls against the rounder side of the uterus. Uterine contractions may aim this breech baby into the right hip, so engagement into the pelvis may take a long while. Sometimes an arm is raised in the left-to-right rotation, and a trained care provider would need to help release the baby.

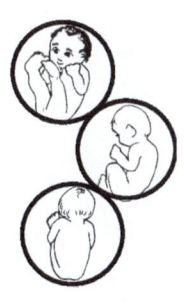

Breech babies turn easier with anatomical space. Create space with body balancing. Breech birth can be safe with a well-trained care provider. Breech birth safety is individual to each birth, baby, parent, and care provider.

© 2025 Restorative Birthwork All rights retained. RestoryBirthwork.com

What If You Find Out Your Baby's Position Isn't Ideal for Birth?

Some head-down positions fit most pelvises more easily than others. Head down is half the story. The term **optimal fetal positioning** (page 73) means positions you do to help baby into an easier position for birth. It's not useful to think in "good" or "bad" positions—or babies! Rather, there is a spectrum of ease (page 70) for all vertical positions. Birthing a baby relies on many variables. If some variables are more ideal (suppleness, pelvic mobility, persistence), they may make up for the less ideal variable of a posterior position or stiffness.

Facing forward, head up, or tipped—baby's position must come to fit the space available. The amazing thing is, you can make more space! Reduce tension in your pelvis by balancing the connecting tissue of your whole anatomy.

A brief, daily home program is usually enough. An appointment with a special bodyworker may be needed by those of us overcoming old falls or chronic pain. Choosing movement, including daily stretches in many directions, is a start.

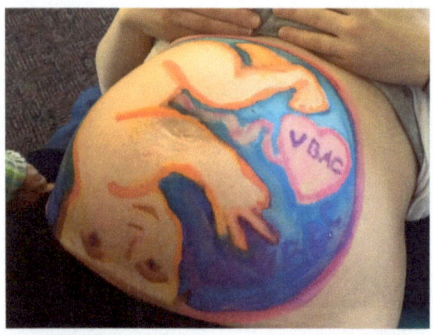

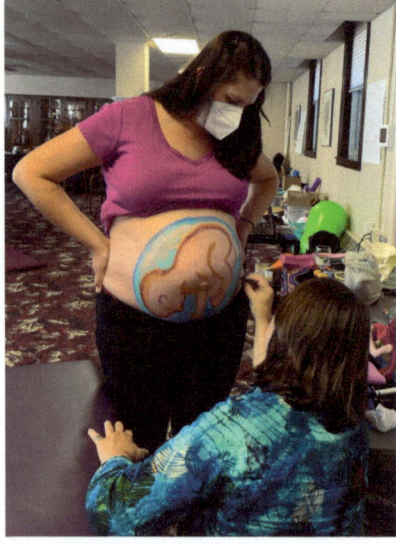

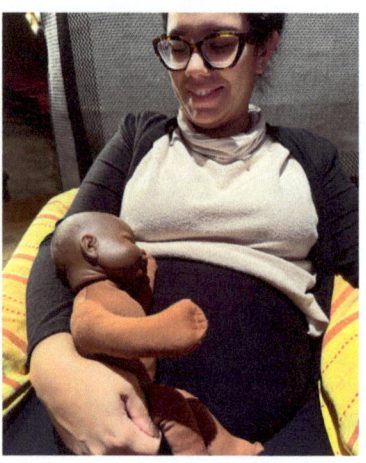

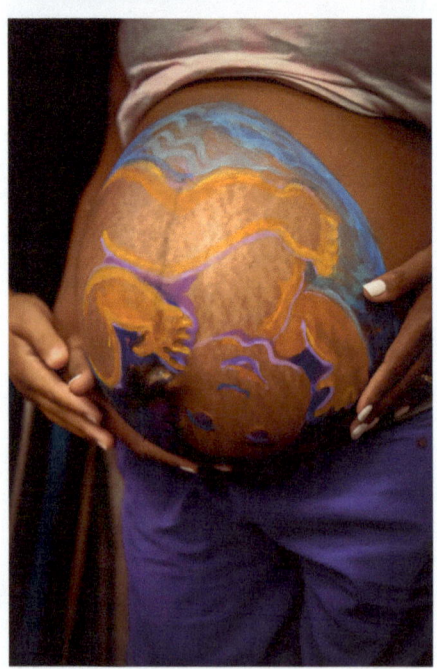

Images on this page, starting at the top left and going clockwise, are:

Right Occiput Posterior with the body transverse; Oblique (Gail painting); Breech (with doll); and Right Occiput Posterior (both hands in front).

Even if baby doesn't change position, your body balancing may help baby have an easier birth than if you didn't activate your *physiology*.

When self-care isn't enough, you might seek professional bodywork or dive deeper into self-care. Resources that you might use are in a section on page 88.

"Babies Can Change Position at Any Time"
There is a position that is the most comfortable for babies: the "fetal position."

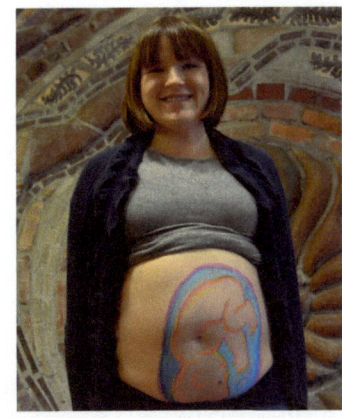

A fetal position is when the entire spine is curled, which tips the chin on the chest. The thighs are flexed near the abdomen. Arms are folded near the chest. Fingers can reach the mouth, letting baby self-comfort and stimulating healthy growth. Baby's gut releases well-being hormones when baby is flexed.

A fetus is neurologically inclined to curl up, which means babies will move into this position when they can. Yet you will hear well-meaning professionals deflect a parent's fear about posterior position by saying, "Some babies are more comfortable in a posterior position." Let's talk about that.

I believe we face fear by sharing practical things we can do, not masking issues. Comfort isn't baby's reason. Here's why: The baby in a right-sided or posterior position has a straight back and lifted chin. An extended posture activates the sympathetic nervous system. Extension is not the classic flexed "fetal position" but rather one of alertness. The trade-off? A super alert baby has more hours to learn!

More babies are posterior today than in the past. Perhaps, as a society, we are more vigilant. The resting and nesting of pregnancy is devalued and interrupted by demands of a fast-paced and sometimes frenetic culture. If the pregnant parent has a very activated sympathetic nervous system, then will the baby be more likely to be in a posterior position? That's a theory that is floating around, if you don't mind the pun.

You may also hear, "Your baby can change position at any time, even in labor." There is truth in that, partially. Contractions turn babies, especially if they've been able to tuck their chins. But which babies are likely to turn and which can't? Would you like to move from chance to self-advocacy for you and your baby?

What Helps a Baby Change Position?
- A uterus in a balanced body—add balance in pregnancy and in labor
- A baby that floats freely in amniotic fluid
- Gravity—yet sleep positions or how you sit are not enough—balance first!
- Powerful contractions
- A balanced womb and pelvis and contractions are likely to help a posterior turn, even with an anterior placenta. Suppleness may make rotation easier

You don't have to leave birth to chance, and you don't have to do this alone.

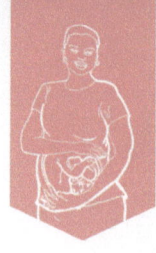

Awakening Inner Wisdom
Nurturing Awareness

Research shows that unborn babies are sentient beings who respond to their parents' emotions, voices, and even thoughts.

Your awareness of your baby as an active participant in your relationship can significantly improve your mental health during pregnancy and strengthen your bond after birth.

The Science Behind Prenatal Connection

A groundbreaking study published in the journal *Mindfulness* followed thirteen mother-baby relationships. The research revealed that women who learned to connect mindfully with their unborn babies experienced:

- Reduced stress, anxiety, and depression during pregnancy
- Better pain management during labor and birth
- Improved breastfeeding experiences
- Stronger feelings of connection with their babies
- Greater confidence in their parenting abilities

This study also found that when parents understand their baby as a sentient being capable of communication, they become more motivated to maintain positive emotional states and make healthier choices throughout pregnancy.

Three Practices for Inner Wisdom

1. **Mindful Baby Communication Practice:** Ask your baby a question and pause to notice movement. Parents report feeling their baby respond with kicks or shifts in position during conversations. Even if you feel like you are "making up" baby's responses, it is valuable and valid to have the *inner* conversations.
2. **Take an Inner Voyage:** With your "mind's eye," look into the womb and either write or draw what you see. Talk to the baby about what it feels like in there, and see if you get any impressions or ideas of your baby's response. Imagine your baby in a very safe and comfortable place, filled with all of the things that you most want to provide.
3. **"Show" Your Baby Something Beautiful:** While seeing something beautiful, cover your eyes with one hand, place the other on your belly, and internally communicate what you have seen. This practice will help you to become more observant, and it is a fun way to connect with your baby.

Creating Your Prenatal Bonding Practice

Five minutes of intentional connection each day makes a significant difference. Approach these practices with curiosity and joy to create the most positive experience for both of you.

Reference

Petersson, M., & Uvnäs-Moberg, K. (2024). Interactions of oxytocin and dopamine—Effects on behavior in health and disease. Biomedicines, 12(11), 2440.

Sansone-Southwood, A., Stapleton, P. B., & Patching, A. (2024). A Qualitative Investigation of a Prenatal Mindfulness Relationship-Based (PMRB) Program to Support Maternal Mental Health and Mother–Baby Relationship During Pregnancy and Post-Partum. *Mindfulness*, 15(7), 1759-1777.

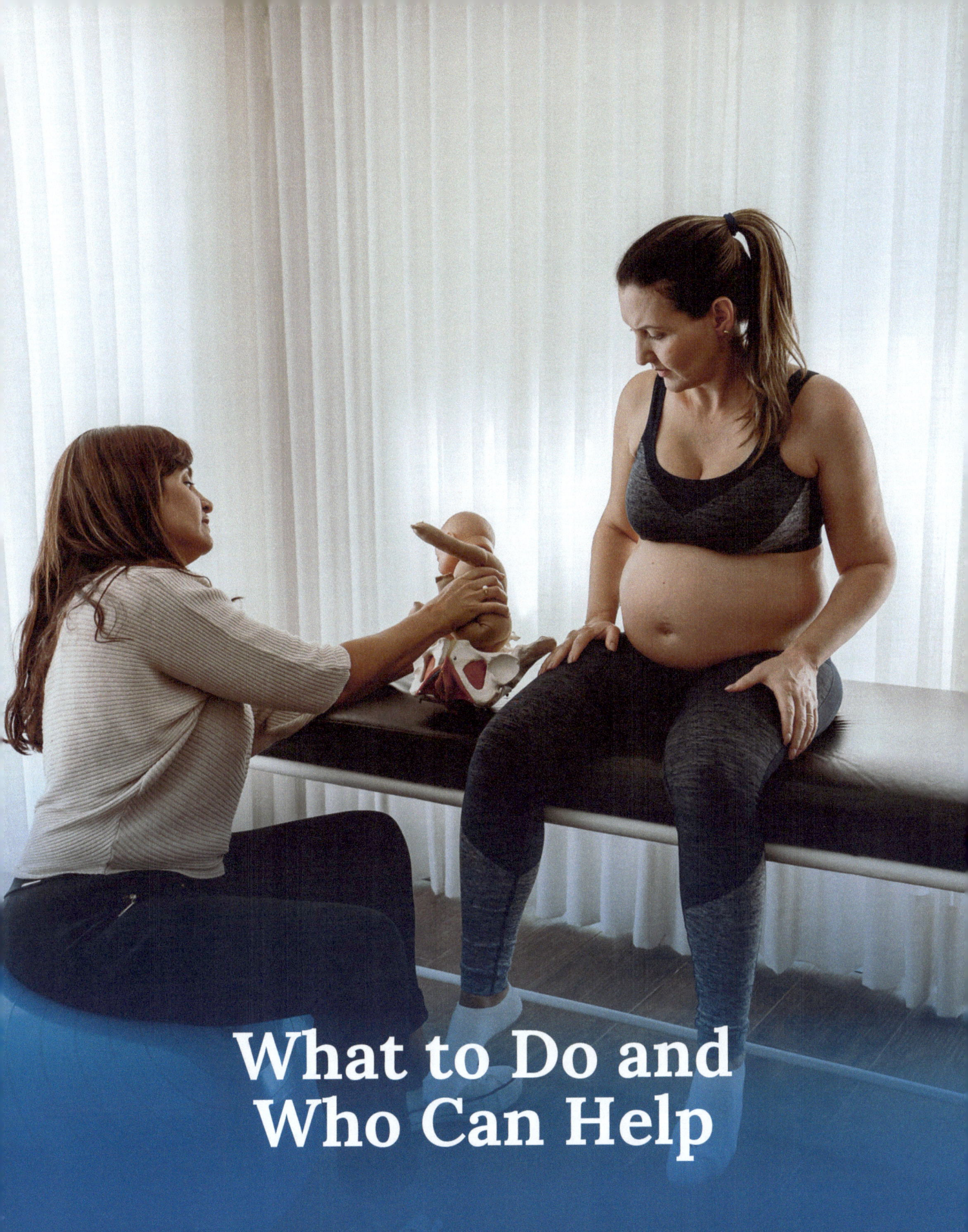

What to Do and Who Can Help

What to Do During Pregnancy

You *can* do a lot to help your baby into position for birth. If your baby is already in the position you hope they stay in, you can still do things we show in three categories to support your pelvis and uterus, which in turn support your baby's position, reduce pain, and ease birth.

You can do this. The following pages invite you to a Spinning Babies® approach.

1. Daily Activities

The first area of birth preparation at Spinning Babies® will free up your range of motion, relaxing your nervous system and lengthening your muscle fibers. We've selected a set of **Daily Activities** to activate the balance you already have available. The care of your body is in your hands. Choose your guide: **website**, **online class**, and especially, with a **Spinning Babies® Certified Parent Educator**.

Walking every day may be the best exercise. To reduce falls and add comfort, stretch daily with pelvis-balancing exercises, such as the triangle pose in yoga, swimming, and dancing. Circle your hips on a firm birth ball around each way.

Left to right below: psoas (*so-as*) lengthening, hip opening, windmills, and anterior pelvic tilts. Not shown: calf stretches, lunges and other activities to mix and match for pelvic flexibility. Gain comfort now and ease during childbirth.

Add poses held in alignment along with slow movement to increase range of motion and support muscle strength. If hypermobile, take care. Core strength is not the goal so much as core suppleness or longer muscles for better function.

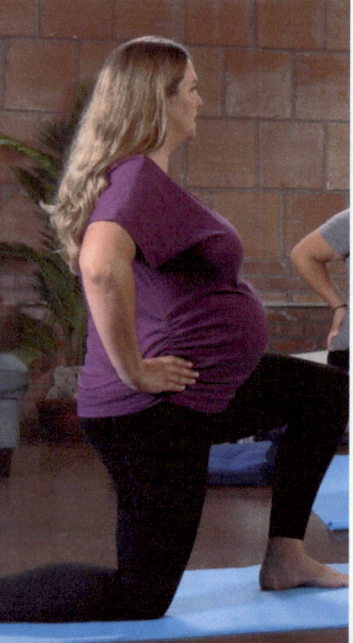 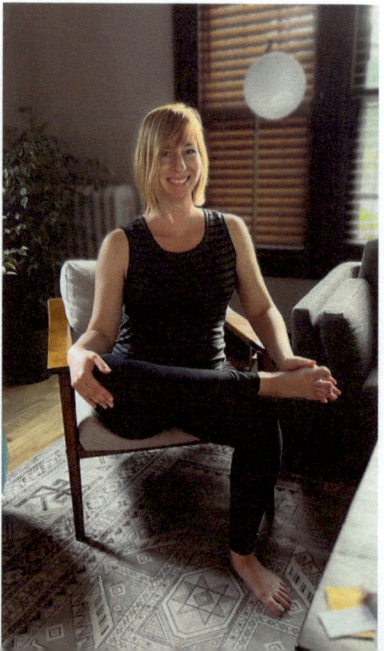 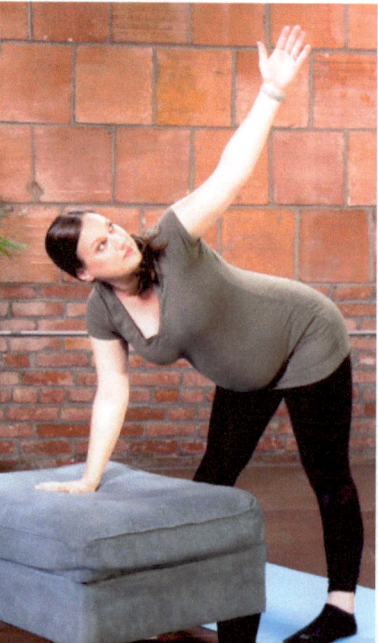 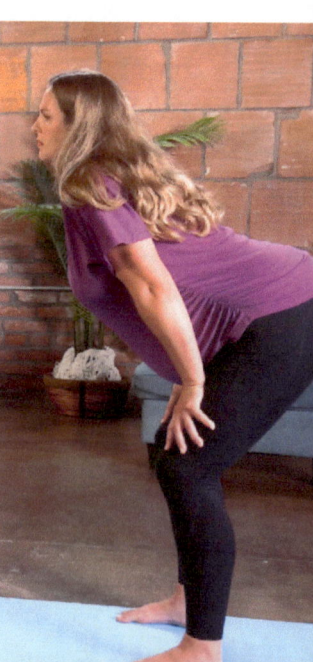

2. Maternal Positioning in Pregnancy

The second area of birth preparation at Spinning Babies® is Move Smart/Rest Smart℠ to preserve the physiology you've activated with Daily Activities.

Move Smart℠

Moving is more than exercise. It's about how we move. Typically, people walk like falling on one foot and then the other, whereas pushing of the back foot and lifting the thigh forward in a long stride is actually restorative. Using proper body mechanics during everyday tasks and props in yoga improves circulation and health.

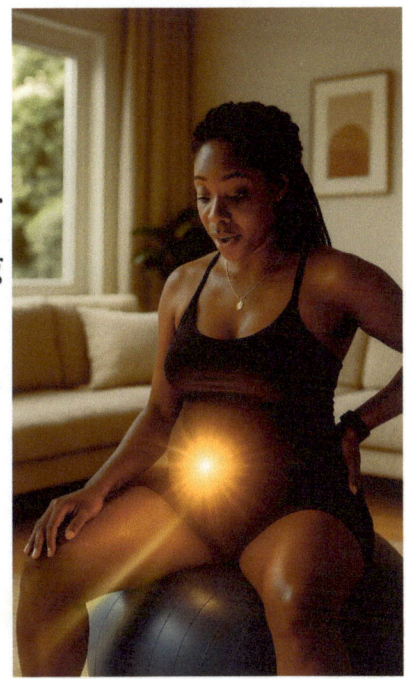

Rest Smart℠

Sit with knees lower than your hips, a tip from Midwife Jean Sutton. This will make your belly a hammock for the baby's back to settle into, as long as there's room. You'll know you have a Rest Smart℠ position when your baby's light shines down (out your navel) toward the earth.

While sleeping or just lying down, support your belly and the small of your back with pillows. A pillow under the top knee and ankle prevents the top leg from hanging and making a twist to **uterine ligaments**. A pillow for your upper arm helps prevent the upper shoulder from falling asleep. Alternate sides according to comfort. Prefer your left side, but accept that you must roll over sometimes!

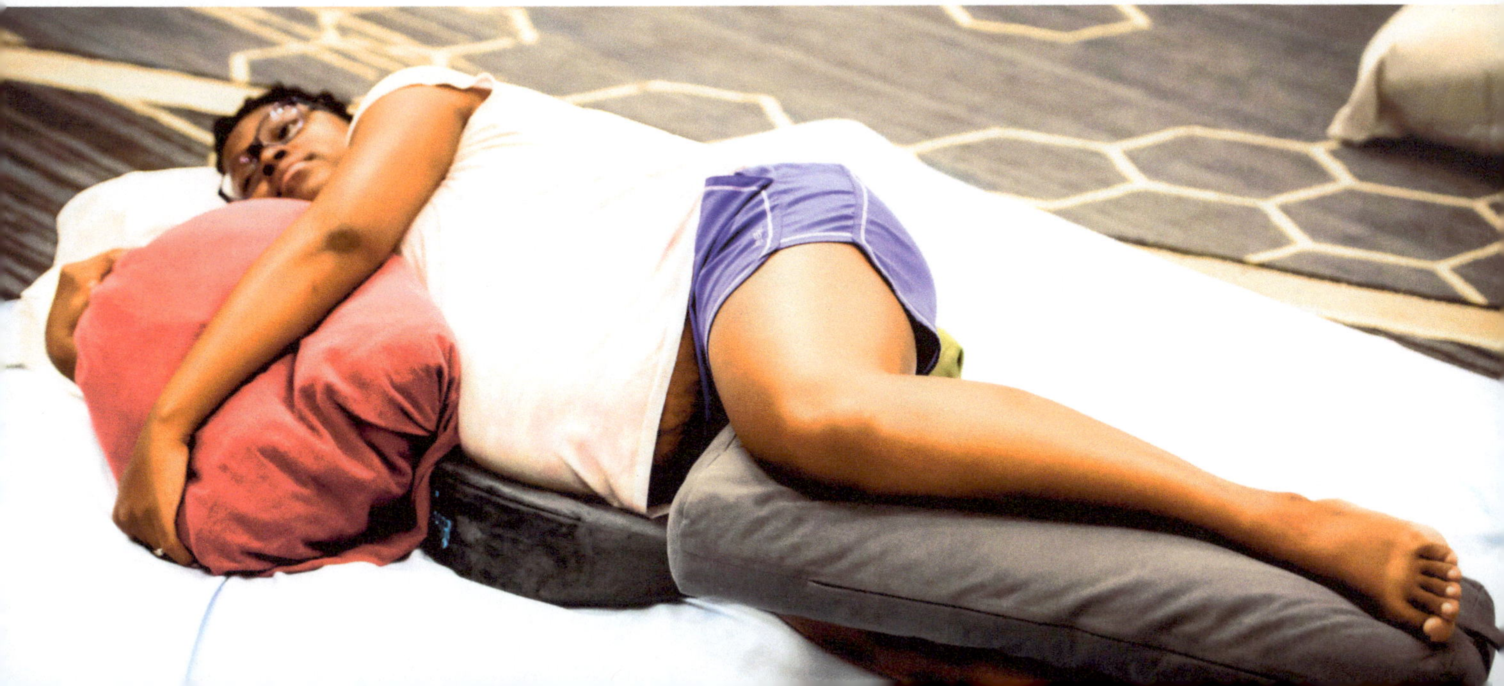

3. Restoring Balance Within the Body

The third area to birth preparation is Spinning Babies® Three Balances℠. Humans have the same ability to reproduce as other mammals. But modern life limits the physicality of the design within. Release your innate birth ability with *body balancing*. Add this advantage to social support and know-how for birth.

Bodywork

Discomfort in pregnancy, including pelvic pain, finding baby's kicks tender, and "*false labor*," can be helped by bodywork. Choose bodywork according to your needs and desires; here are major modalities that we like:

- Chiropractic
- Osteopathic
- *Craniosacral therapy*
- Spinning Babies® Aware Practitioner
- Dynamic Body Balancing™
- Fasciatherapy (Danis Bois Method)
- Ortho-Bionomy
- *Maya uterine massage*
- Rebozo manteada
- Acupuncture
- *Moxibustion*
- *Homeopathy*

Body Balancing Can Be Added to or Part of Any Bodywork

Not all bodywork is body balancing. Relaxation massage will calm your nervous system, but it won't balance the tensions of the body. Where chronic stiffness or tension exists, *fascial release*/therapy and/or unwinding will improve all others.

Balance in the body optimizes coping, timing and length of labor, stretching to open the cervix and perineum, and recovery.

If you can't find or afford soft-tissue body balancing locally, you can do self-care with the Three Balances℠ (shown below) and other releases. To get the how-to, we refer you to our website and to a Spinning Babies® Certified Parent Educator.

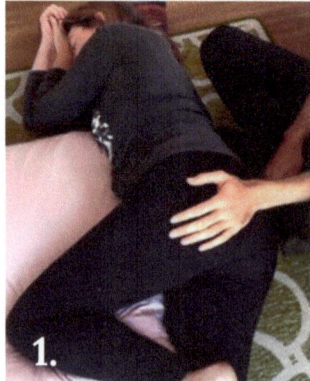
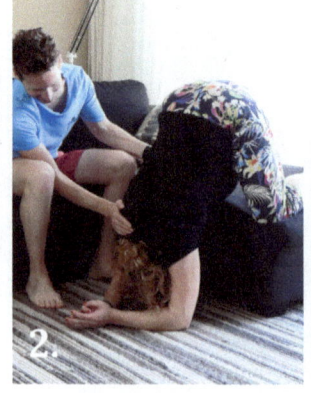
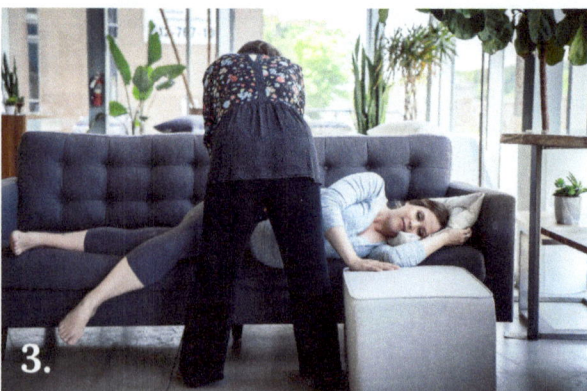

The Jiggle creates a deep relaxation.

Forward-leaning Inversion (FLI) is a reset.

Side-lying Release (SLR) is a slow, static stretch that may help align baby and pelvis.

Restoring the Innate Balance Waiting Inside Your Body
The human body is a structure held together by the pull of connective tissues. If a muscle or **ligament** is pulled stronger than its partner can match, the body is pulled out of balance. Tension imbalances can happen from repetitive activity of the same sport or job, from a fall, or just from years of being in gravity, especially when on the couch. We all experience varying effects on parts of our bodies.

You may need more than a comprehensive stretching or yoga routine if there is pain, trouble walking, discomfort sitting or sleeping, or a fetal position that won't fit the pelvis.

Balancing the tensions or twists in the uterine ligaments or pelvis and back may bring a great deal of comfort and perhaps a more birth-friendly fetal position.

Breathing Is Balancing
Deep and slow breathing is not just for calming. Breathing deep and slow builds and releases internal body pressure and massages your organs for renewal.

Breathing to expand your lungs bottom-to-top and side-to-side during quiet times and with exercise movements changes the pressures inside the body to help circulation and massage organs.

> "Each contraction brings you closer to your baby and your baby closer to you." —Penny Simkin

Letting Labor Begin on Its Own
Research studies support the **spontaneous onset of labor**. If your caregiver does suggest induction, ask whether this is based on medical needs or usual care. For some, the advantages of induction will reduce the risks of a medical condition. Body balancing and smarter birth positions may support your sense of control in an induced labor, as well as help line up baby and release true oxytocin.

Imagining Labor as Friendly
Labor has a purpose besides letting your baby through your body. The oxytocin released in "**natural birth**" gives actual pain relief, making you a little high, sleepy, and wanting to see your baby. Contractions also turn babies who are flexed.

Dr. Michel Odent recommends dim lights, privacy, quiet murmurs or music, and sometimes silence to support the hormones of birthing. Let go of "doing things right" to be present with what you feel in your body, and respond instinctively.

Even pleasure is possible in birthing.

Support in Pregnancy Is Support for Life

Find Birth Support Now
Gather your own circle of support. Whether you have loved ones and community or you join a group, social support during pregnancy is proven to improve your experience and your baby's health!

Childbirth classes are a way to meet other parents. Spinning Babies® certifies childbirth educators to guide parents through important techniques and new birth positions for easier childbirth. Imagine a **Spinning Babies® Certified Educator** showing your birth partner just the right way to support you to bring comfort right now and help your birth be more comfortable.

The continuous presence of a birth ***doula*** from early labor is proven to raise birth satisfaction, even for the partner! A nonrelated, nonmedical person who knows birth and puts your emotional needs first actually reduces complications and the sensation of pain. Doula care is not just a "feel-good" luxury. Find doulas online at www.dona.org or do an online search for local doula organizations.

Nutritional Support
A healthy baby grows from the healthy foods you eat right now. Everyone wants a treat once in a while. But to keep things in balance, eat healthy food first. Five servings of vegetables to one carb serving. Eat six servings of protein each day (an example of one day's protein: two eggs, a cup of yogurt, a piece of cheese, 4 Tbsp of almond butter on an apple, half a chicken breast, and a handful of nuts). Choose fruit instead of fruit juice. Don't avoid all salt. Drink 3-4 qts of water.

Mental Health
Our physical, emotional, spiritual, and mental health are also quadrants of a whole. They work together. When one quadrant is expressing unmet needs, a crisis can affect the whole. Our mental health is key to how we see ourselves, our world, and our babies. Times of change, like birth, accentuate a sense of the unknown. Our mind will make stories to find stability, and our stories match our physiology. By activating our parasympathetic nervous system, we increase calm and resilient stories to interpret our lives and others. Our babies grow well when the hormones released with the parasympathetics include a sense of well-being for us and our babies. This is one way we are able to access our inner wisdom.

Professional counseling or therapy can be vital. NAMI is a national source with chapters in many states—**www.nami.org/your-journey/maternal-new-parent-mental-health/mental-health-during-pregnancy**.

Games to Play with Your Baby

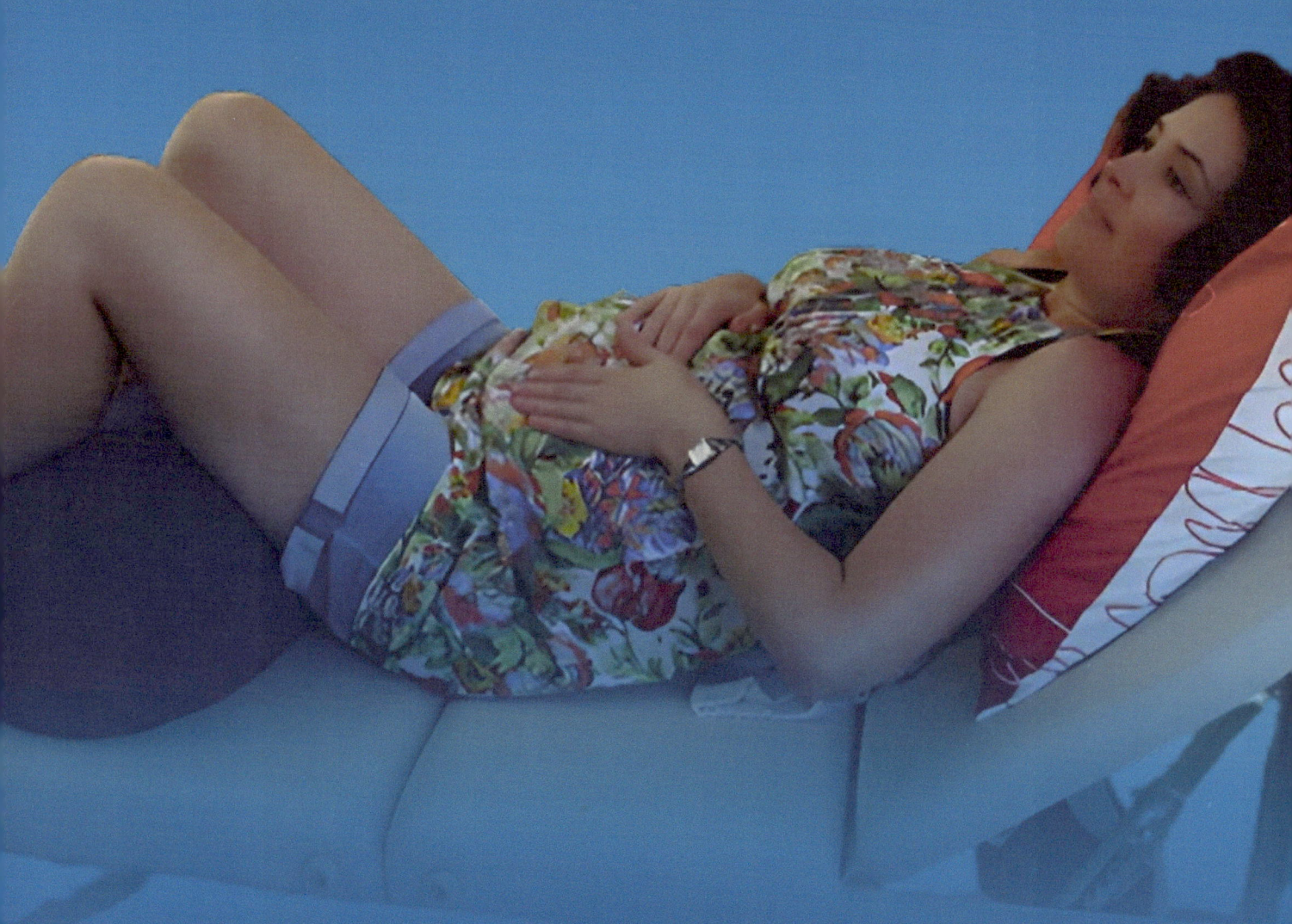

Games to Play with Your Baby

As you settle in to feel the shapes of your baby's body each day, linger and enjoy the fact that your baby is aware of you. Babies are incapable of judgment. They accept and love readily.

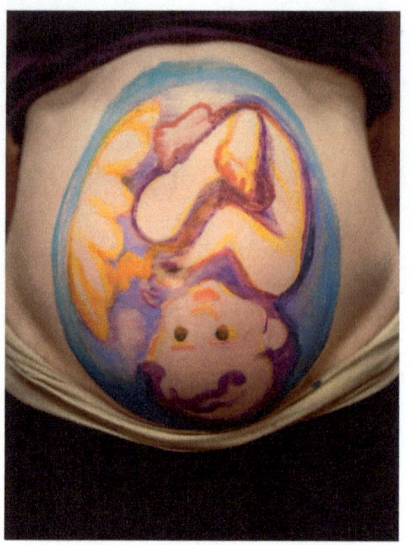

In the ups and downs of human existence, one of the most beautiful expressions of life is your relationship together—so much so that there is a special word for it, *Mamatoto*, or MotherBaby.

Gestation develops a baby but can also develop a loving parent. Whether you identify as mother or other, the heart of this connection invites an archetypal symbology you can claim for your own.

Breathing Waves of Love

HeartMath Institute and others show consistent data that the heart and brain generate coherent wave patterns after several minutes of a breathing style.

Settle into a semi-reclining position. Begin to settle your breath. Just breathe naturally at first. Gradually begin to slow your breath. It's OK if you fall asleep!

1. Breathe in for both of you. Let your baby know the heart of you as a loving, welcoming presence. Exhale for both of you.
2. Now, focus on your heart. Imagine breathing in and out of your heart.
3. Learn to match the time it takes to breathe in with the time it takes to breathe out. Inhale and exhale with the same 5- or 6-second intervals.
4. With practice, learn to move the same amount of air in and out with smooth transitions from inhaling to exhaling "through the heart."
5. Add a heart-centered emotion, like gratitude, welcome, or love. Sustain any joyful or beneficent emotion (illustration).

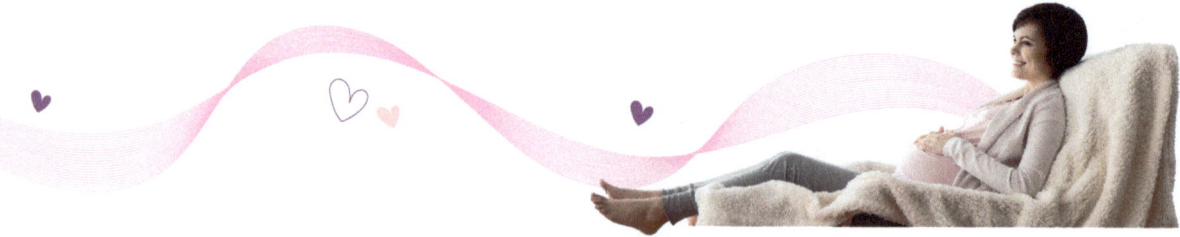

Breathing wave-like and radiating love help baby regulate their emotions, too.

Reference
Poston, P. D. (2017). Change of heart: An integral inquiry into prenatal depression, heartmath, and transformation. [Doctoral dissertation, Sofia University].

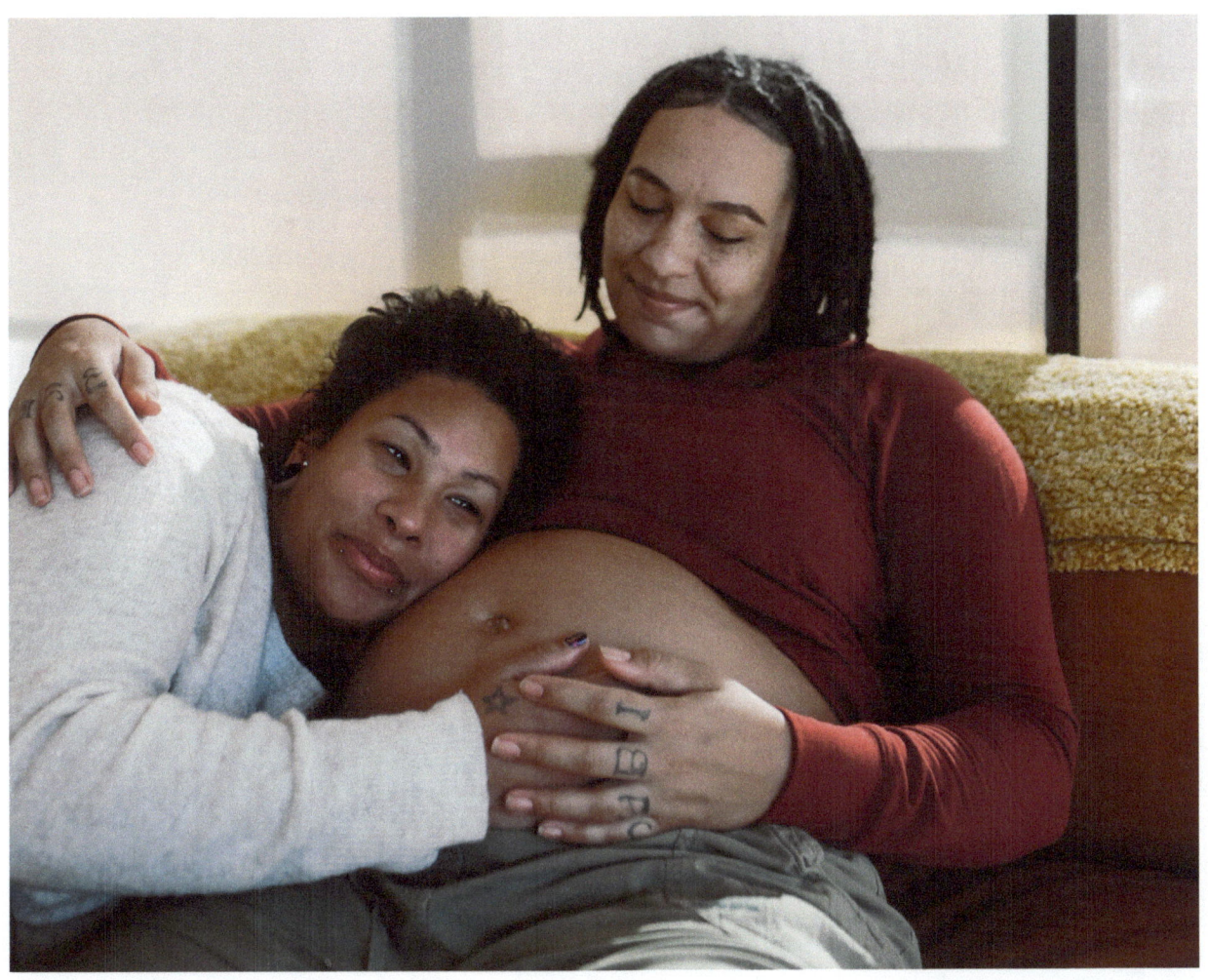

Follow the Light
Here's an idea some of us midwives and doulas have had to encourage baby into position. Shine a flashlight on the lower abdomen on the right side. We think that when there is easy room for baby to turn themselves, babies may look at the faint glow made by a strong flashlight.

Before birth, a strong light becomes a soft orange light through the layers of the abdomen. We would never shine such a light directly into anyone's eyes after they were born.

Play this game after doing a body-balancing routine in pregnancy, such as from Spinning Babies® or after getting bodywork, when the ligaments are softer and easier for baby to turn past. The hope is a baby turns their back to the left to look at the light. Since a light won't shine through a spine, the right side will do.

The Kick Game

Researchers followed several fathers playing a regular game of "Tap." Each evening, your partner, baby's father or other parent, might slowly and rhythmically press into your belly near the baby's hands or feet and say out loud, "Tap!" or "Let's play!"

Babies process rather slowly, so wait six full seconds before you tap again. Repeat six times each night. See how many nights it takes for baby to tap back! Play often and play slowly.

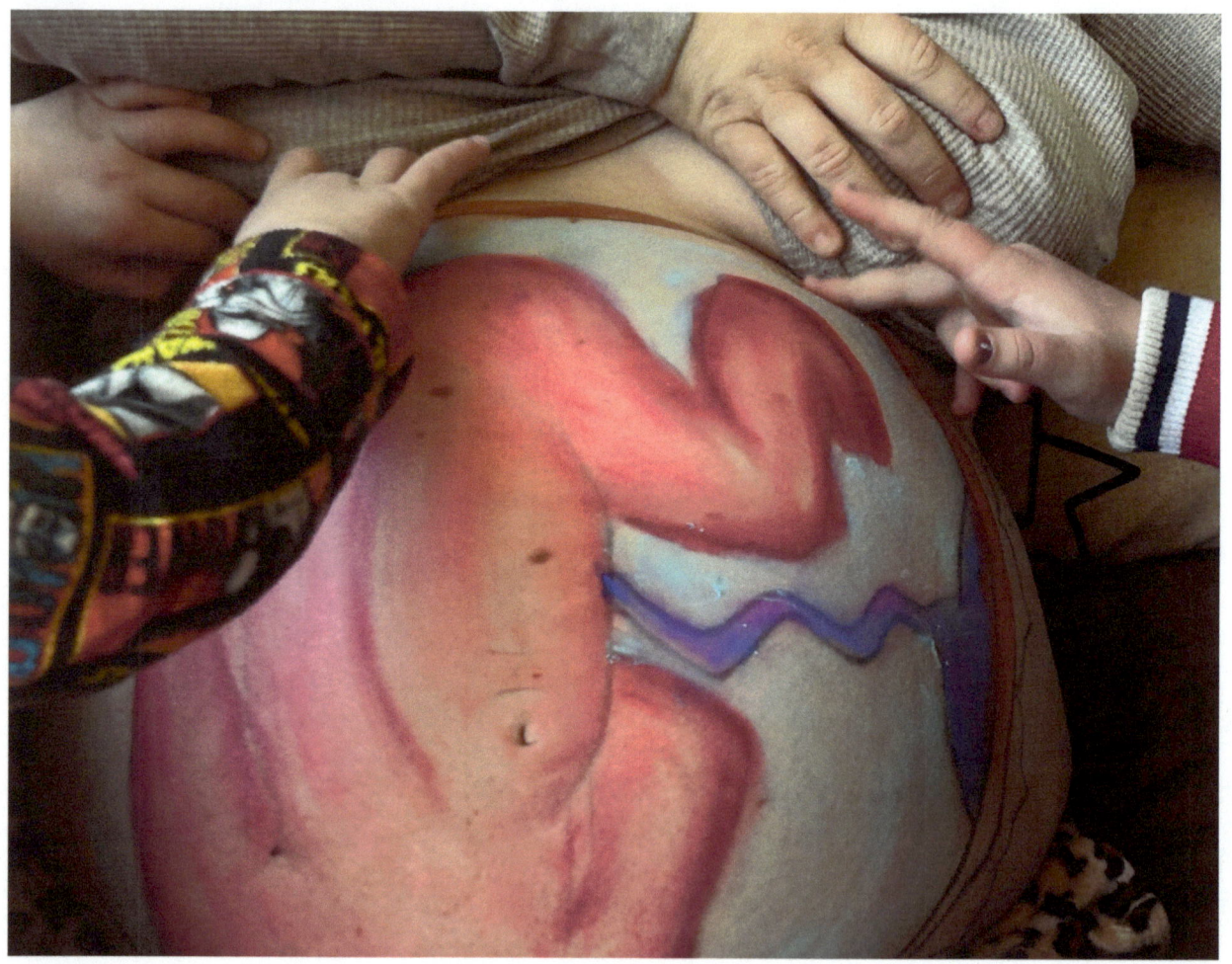

References
1. Kenner, C., & Lubbe, W. (2007). Fetal stimulation—a preventative therapy. *Newborn and Infant Nursing Reviews, 7*(4), 227-230. https://doi.org/10.1053/j.nainr.2007.06.013
2. Schwartzenberger, K. (2020). Neurosensory play in the infant-parent dyad: A developmental perspective. In *Infant Play Therapy* (pp. 37-49). Routledge.
3. Van de Carr, F. R. (1988). Prenatal university: Commitment to fetal-family bonding and the strengthening of the family unit as an educational institution. *Journal of Prenatal & Perinatal Psychology & Health, 3*(2), 87.

Singing

Sing a song. Research shows babies remember music and singing. The voices of loved ones are heard in the womb from early gestation. Before 17 weeks after conception, which is 15 weeks of gestation, a baby begins to hear. Singing the same happy song each day becomes a familiar reassurance for the growing fetus.

Then, after birth, singing that same song has been shown to calm them, reducing stress chemicals in their blood and improving heart rate and other vital physiological functions.

Singing connects us to creative centers in the brain, expanding intelligence beyond the factual left hemisphere into arts and language, including the language of mathematics.

References
1. Adachi, M., & Trehub, S. E. (2012). Musical lives of infants. In G. McPherson & G. Welch (Eds.), *The Oxford handbook of music education* (pp. 229-247). New York: Oxford Uni Press.
2. Simkin, P. (2013). Singing to The Baby. https://youtu.be/gsdEK6OxucA?si=9wm8gywBX9weetxN
3. Chamberlain, D. (2013). *Windows to the womb*. North Atlantic Books.

Dancing Touch

Babies move their arms "with" you. I don't mean imitate, but I do mean they join you when you rub your belly. Babies move their hands and arms and heads in response to touches on the belly. Here's a game to activate this knowledge:

Play Beethoven or Mozart (babies seem to like the coherent classics best, but a waltz or lullaby is also heart coherent). Find something you like and play it. Don't play it louder than you would if your baby were outside the womb.

Rub your belly in time with the music. With massage-like strokes, lift up from the sides three times in a row (stroke forward if you are standing!), then stroke up from the bottom three times. Finally, rub a circle from your bottom right side up over your womb and down the left side (like a rainbow). Repeat.

What about just dancing? Yes, Perjés found that prenatal dance benefited those fetuses when they were toddlers with better memory.

References
1. Perjés, B. B. (2023). Effects of a special prenatal dance method on fetal and postnatal neurodevelopment, maternal physical, psychological, cognitive, social wellbeing, and childbirth [Doctoral dissertation, University of Pécs].
2. Marx, V., & Nagy, E. (2015). Fetal behavioural responses to maternal voice and touch. PLOS One, 10(6), e0129118. https://doi.org/10.1371/journal.pone.0129118

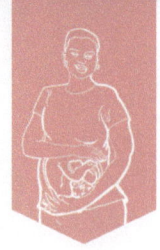

Inviting Bliss
Early Programming for Lifelong Outcomes

Research shows that the prenatal period is crucial for laying the foundation of a child's future success. During pregnancy, the baby develops early mental processes that influence future relationships, stress responses, and cognitive skills.

Biological Benefits of Secure Prenatal Attachment
- Better stress regulation across the lifespan
- Positive genetic expression influenced by maternal mental health
- Epigenetic changes enhancing resilience and emotional regulation
- Lifelong impact on career and relationship quality

Cognitive Advantages of Secure Attachment
- Improved memory formation and retention from birth
- Enhanced ability to anticipate and adapt to the environment
- Greater social understanding and empathy
- Stronger capacity to learn and adjust

Long-Term Outcomes
Children with secure prenatal attachment tend to:
- Excel academically and professionally
- Maintain stable, healthy relationships
- Demonstrate leadership, creativity, and innovation
- Enjoy better physical health and moral reasoning
- Experience higher life satisfaction and happiness

Three Practices to Enhance Prenatal Attachment
1. **Create a Special Spot**—Dedicate a comfortable space to reflect on your baby's future, adding comforting elements like a candle or flowers.
2. **Prepare the Baby's Things**—Treat preparing clothing and nursery items as welcoming a cherished guest.
3. **Gather Blessings**—Collect wishes and blessings from family and friends in a special place to feel your community's support.

Implications for Our Future
For expectant parents, nurturing mental health and bonding during pregnancy is key to fostering lifelong well-being. For society, supporting pregnant families through health and social services is a cost-effective investment in collective success. Prenatal attachment strongly predicts academic, career, relational, and overall life achievements, highlighting its transformative potential.

Reference
Santaguida, E., & Bergamasco, M. (2024). A perspective-based analysis of attachment from prenatal period to second year postnatal life. *Frontiers in Psychology, 15*, 1296242. https://doi.org/10.3389/fpsyg.2024.1296242

BELLY PAINTING
Bonus Section

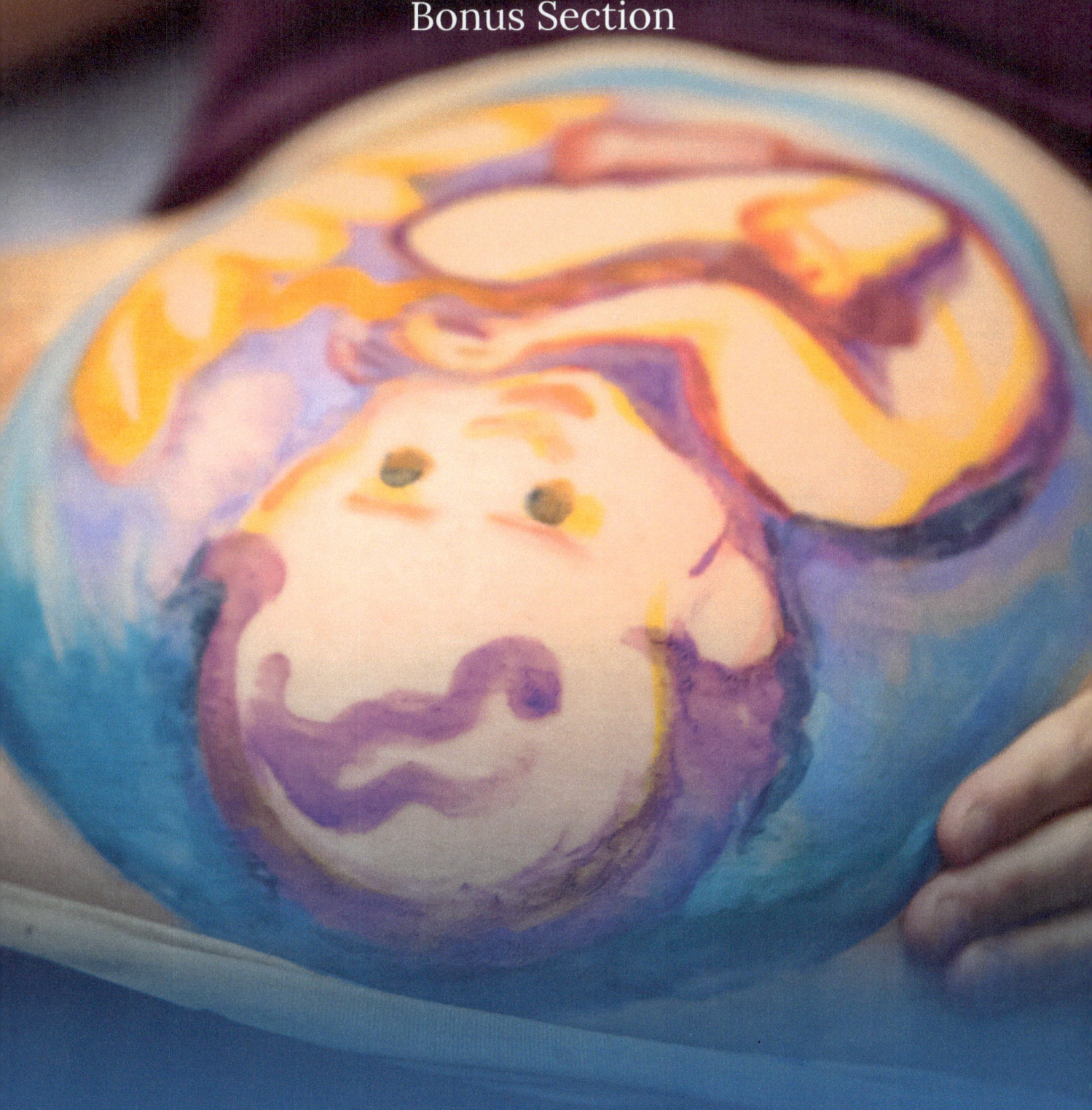

The Benefits of Painting Pregnant Bellies!

Painting a pregnant belly is joyful and fun for everyone. The belly-painting process invites the celebration of pregnancy with self, family, and friends! This is a wonderful way of welcoming baby in a shared bonding event.

This part is written for a painter, not the pregnant person. Belly painting presents an option for Step 2 of The Belly Mapping® Method.

A Prenatal Bonding Opportunity
Your image invites the expression of feelings about the baby. Take a moment to pre-design your picture to inspire connection and joy by the parent(s) and all.

Your Words Invite Feelings About Oneself
Your choice of words, tone of voice, breathing, and facial expressions can create a safe social experience. The painter uses the art of words, as well as the medium of painting, to enhance a feeling that a baby is cherished. Love is there, but the art magnifies the love. The painter sets the mood for love and joy in this magical process of revealing a baby through art.

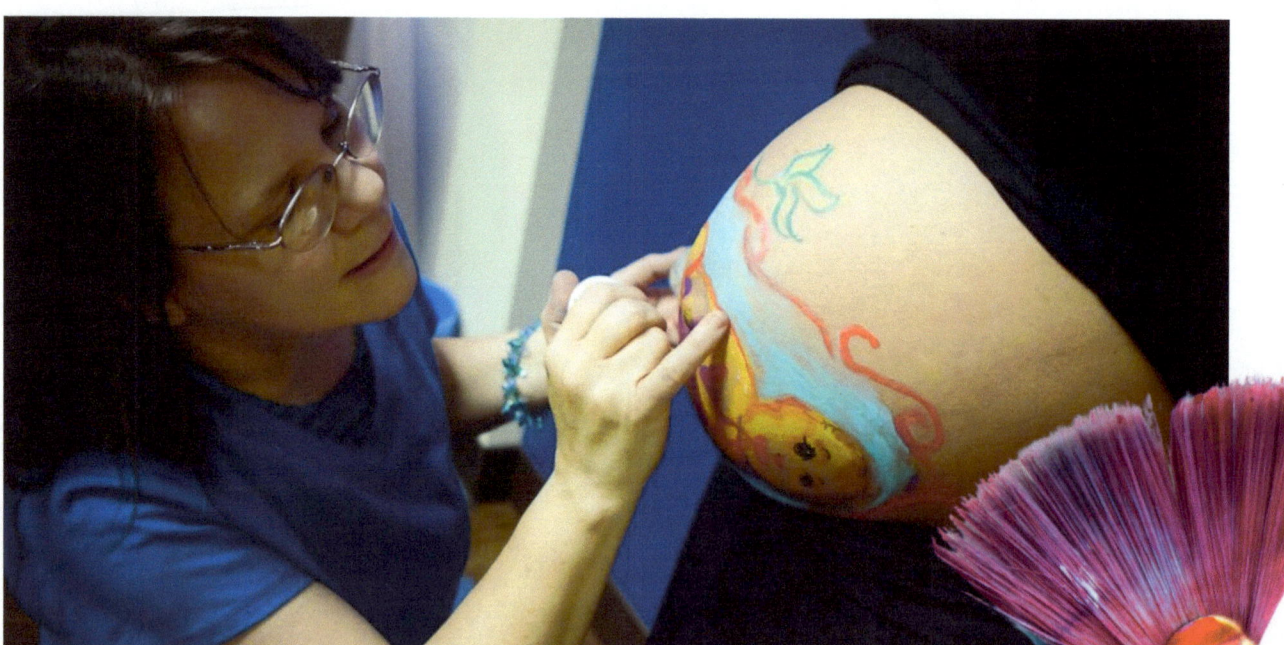

Pregnant women express delight when they see their painting, especially in sharing such delight with loved ones.

This joy is more than a great feeling. You're creating an opportunity for a rare and unique "visit" with their prenatal baby!

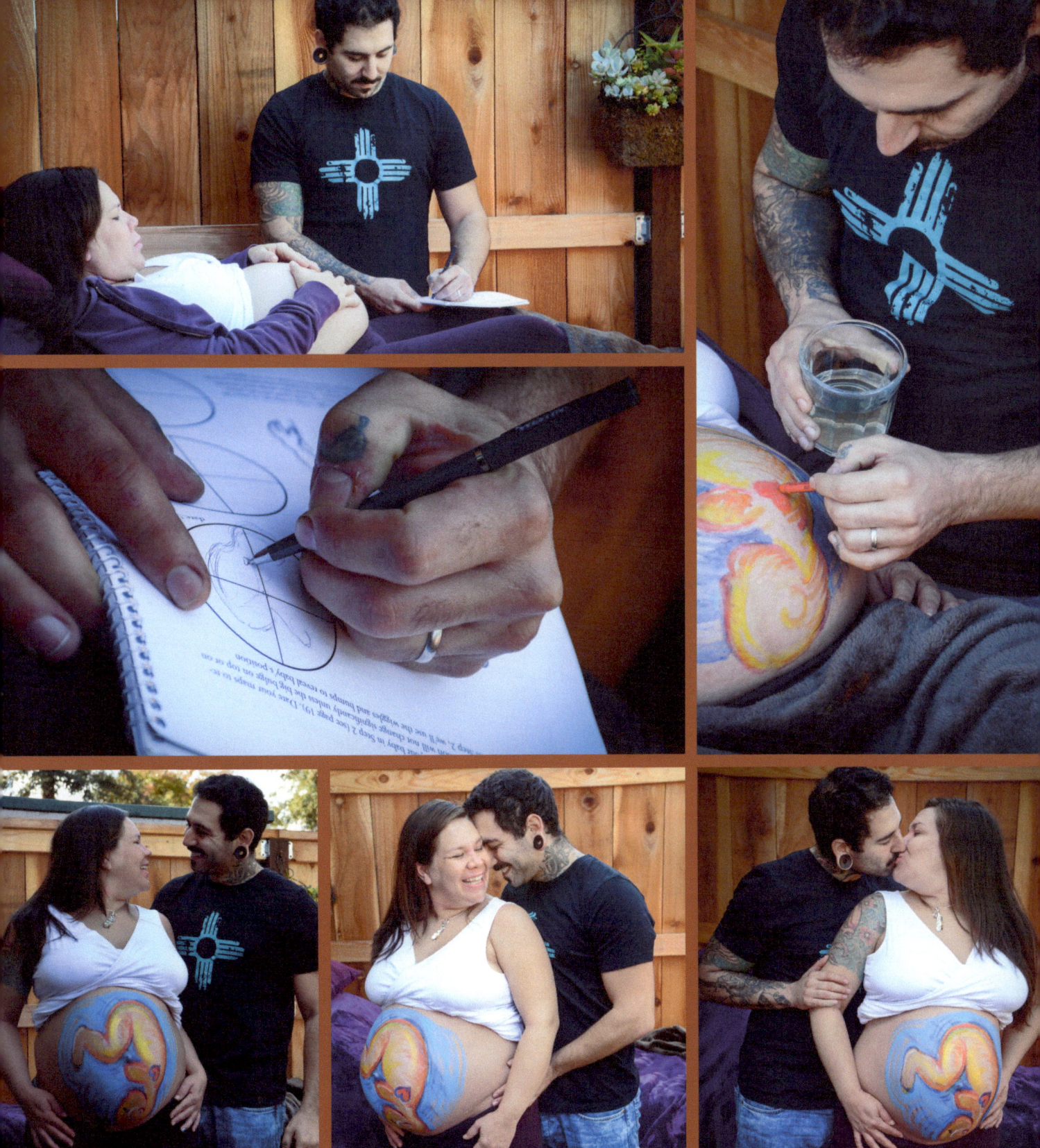

Cassandra and Daniel Dagones
Bond Over The Belly Mapping® Method

Before You Begin

Practice
A round belly is not a flat canvas! The perspective will be convex, like the back of a spoon, not like on flat paper.

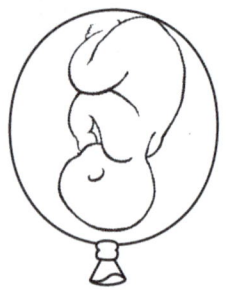

Practice on a balloon or round fruit or vegetable.
A permanent marker is appropriate for an inert object, like a balloon. A nontoxic marker, crayon, or paint is for people.

Are You Using the Map or Palpating the Baby?
You can use the mother's map from their Belly Mapping® Method session as your guide and copy baby's position. If using the map, the pregnant person could sit or stand for the entire painting. If it helps, perhaps draw the baby on paper first as a guide for the final belly drawing.

If the mother is interested in letting you feel the baby so you can "trace" the baby on the abdomen, she'll lie on a couch or massage table. The painter will feel the baby's contours to get a sense of the back, shoulder, buttocks, and limbs.

Note the angle of baby's back, the locations of the kicks, and where the shoulder is to help you estimate the fetal position. Then mentally raise all the parts so you can include the head where it will be visible.

Refer to the sensation map or Fetal Compass Rose in the main portion of this book as a guideline to a fetal position. Whether or not the exact position is matched in your art, the most important thing is creating another channel for bonding to the baby within.

Decisions About Drawing the Baby's Position
Most parents will be happy if you paint (or draw) the baby in the position they are currently in. However, some parents prefer to have their baby drawn in an optimal starting position for birth to help them visualize the baby in the position they hope baby will be in. Decide the position of your portrait with the parent(s) before you begin.

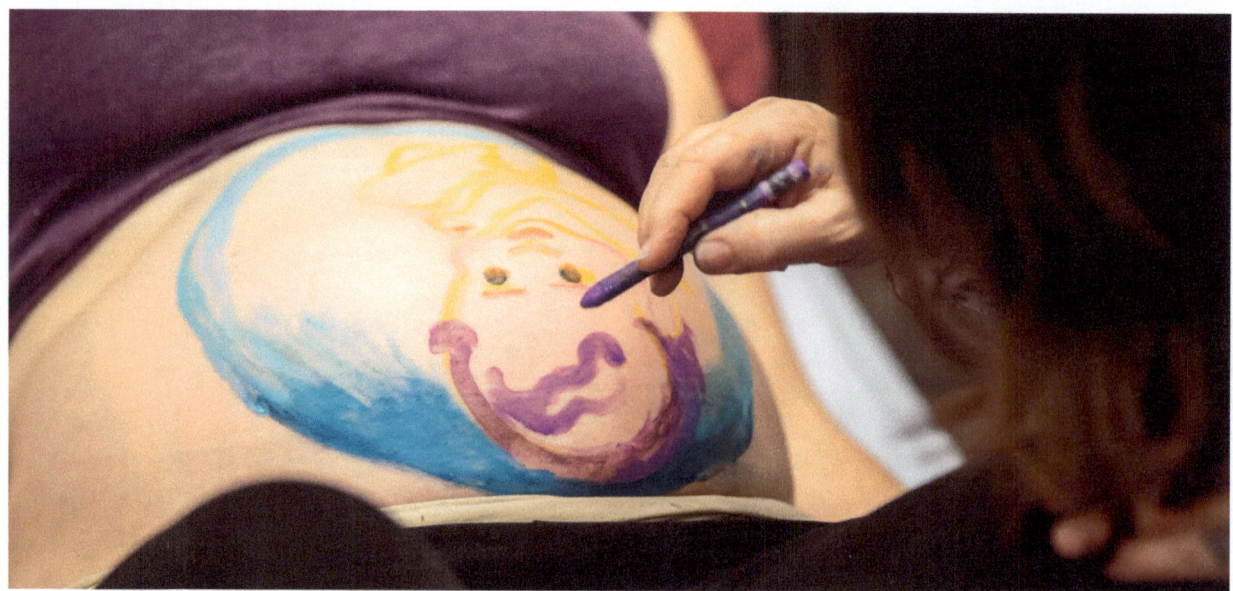

Materials

You can choose water-soluble crayons, **nontoxic markers**, or high-quality **nontoxic face paints**. Note that cheap pigments often include lead or other heavy metals that are not declared on packaging.

A company that claims natural pigments is **Natural Earth Paint**. I've been using nontoxic **Caran d'Ache Neocolor II Aquarelle Artists' Crayons**. Wolfe Colors are the most common professional face and body paints.

- Crayons, markers, or paint
- Bowl of water
- **Paintbrushes, natural or other soft bristle**
- Soft thin cloth, soft tissues, paper towels to dab drips
- A tray with edges to hold materials and to catch spilled fluids
- Couch, massage table, or bed, and pillows for head and knees.

Tips: Solid blocks of color look streaky on a photo, so create with strokes in mind. Dip the crayons in water and let them sit a moment before painting for best results. Professional paintbrushes will make a better picture.

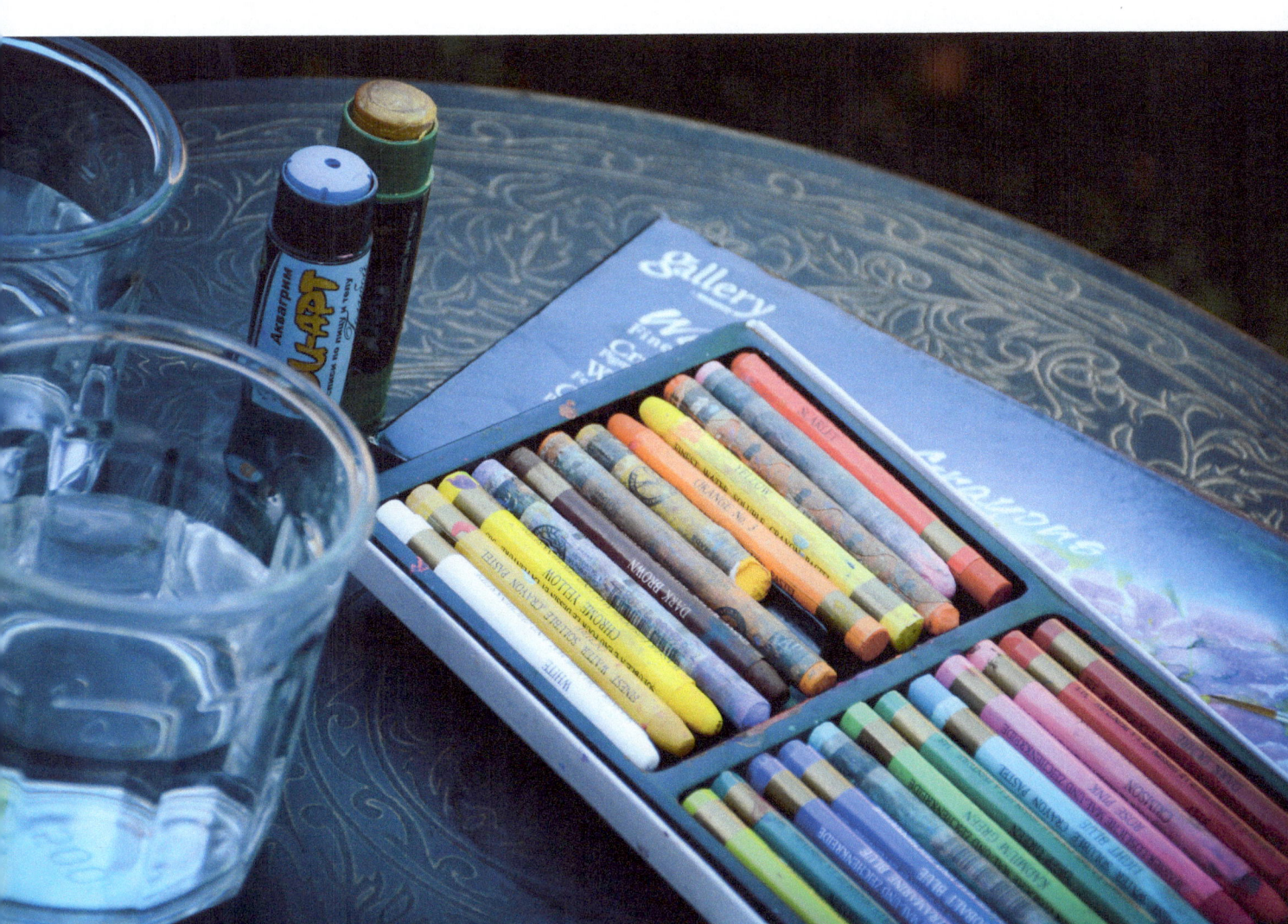

Select Your Colors

Complement skin color, clothing colors, and preferences. Choose whether you will draw three layers, or three layers plus an outline, or a single color for a line drawing. If more than one color, choose a variety of light and dark colors for depth and interest.

The first layer of three layers will be a color close to the skin color of your subject. This is the sketch of the baby. The lack of contrast helps with erasures and redraws.

The second layer of the body is the luminous layer (if you want one). A pale yellow, orange, or a pale pink for pale skin, a light red violet for melanated skin.

The third layer is the final color. This color can be realistic or a bright version complementing the mother's skin color and/or clothes. This layer complements the second layer.

Once you are content with your sketch, you will draw over your sketch with a second layer of color for luminosity to help the third layer on top be most vivid.

Resist the urge to draw dark or bold until you have these two underlying layers. This is hard to resist, but will make your image "cleaner" and dramatic.

You can also draw a single layer in a color that is easy to see.

Create a Sketch Beneath

Without worrying about commitment to the drawing, begin with a light sketch of the entire baby, but not the face, fingers, or toes. This first layer will "fade" into the background after painting a more visible layer on top of it. You can make changes easily before adding brighter or darker colors.

We discuss adding more color layers and details next.

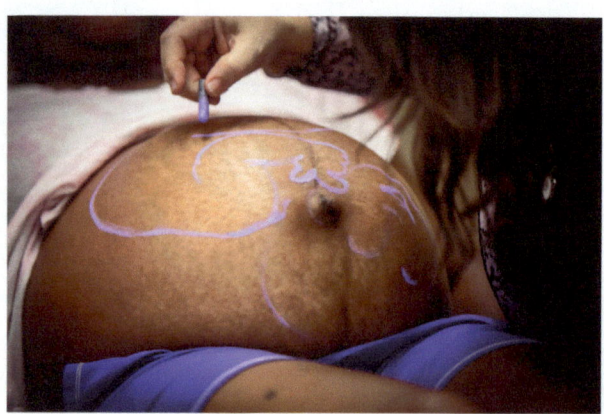
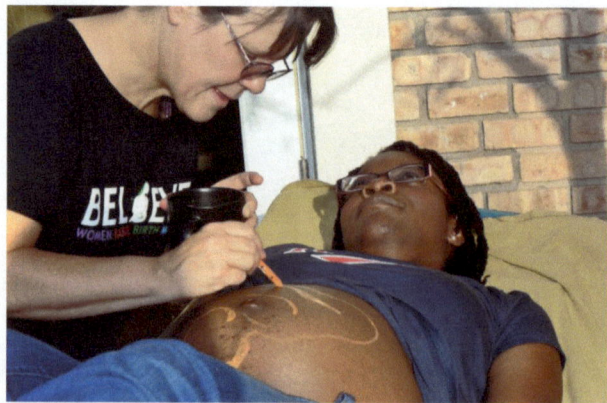

Baby Parts to Paint

Drawing the Head.
The head is one-third of the total length of the head and torso combined. Remember the legs are folded up. Draw the size of the head so that the body can be twice as long and still fit the belly. The back of the head will be bigger than you can feel it. The ear is closer to the face than an adult's. The eye is the same height as the ear.

For bonding joys, you'll want to give baby a head that can be seen! Draw the top of the head, and any hair so it's visible, though the mother needs the help of a camera!

Get a sense of whether the head faces forward, backward, or to the side. The baby will face opposite its back.

Decide whether you are going to draw baby's face now so you know which way the head will face. But wait to draw the face until the background color (or outline) for the face has dried.

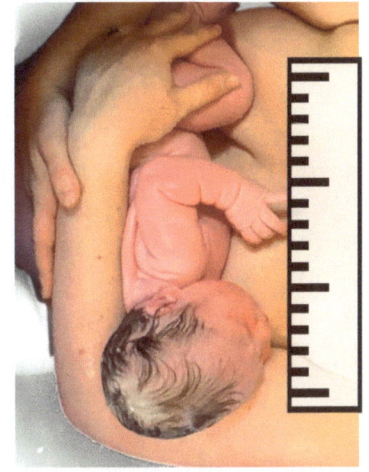

I've tipped the photo on its side so it's easier to see the ratio of head to body as you'll draw the baby. The head and the mother's hand are about ⅓ the length of the body (before the legs). Use your hand as an aid in measuring your drawing.

 Some mothers, while wanting the picture, could find beginning with their lower belly a bit intimate and may feel more comfortable if you start higher on their belly.

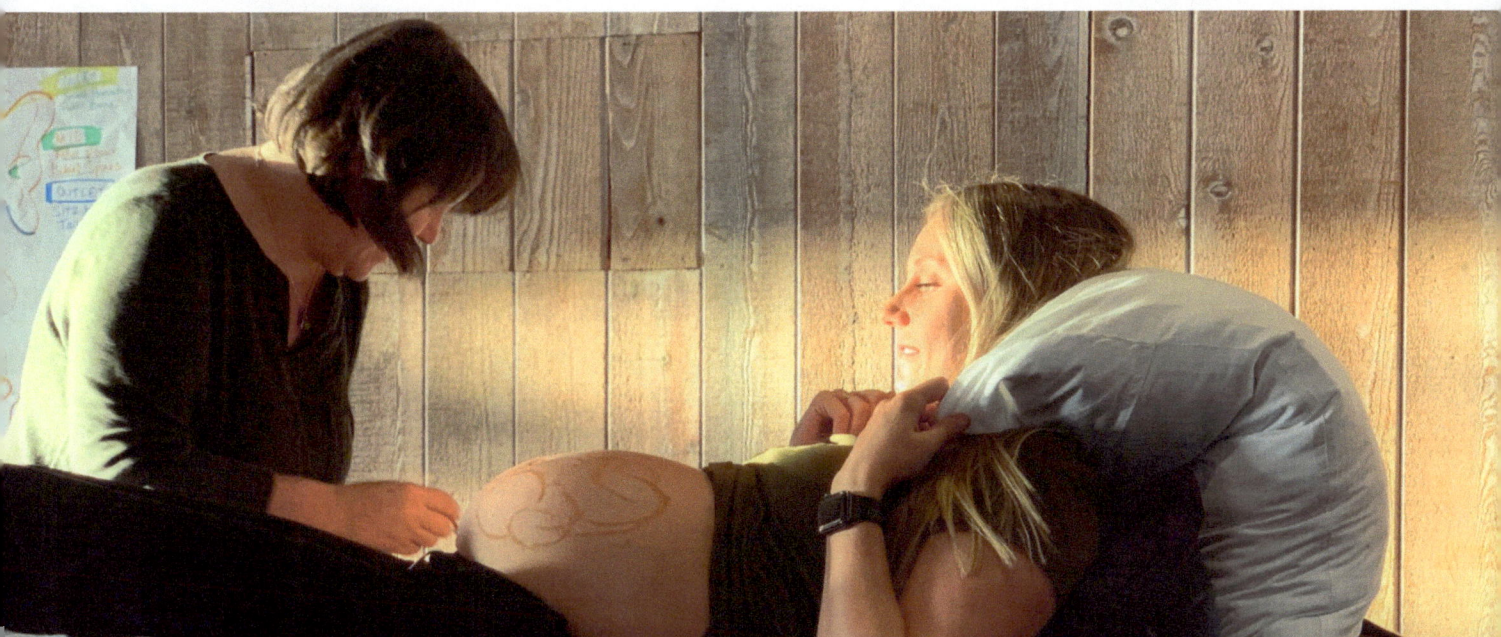

Drawing the Body

While I feel for the location of the back and buttocks, I will "raise them up" in my sketch to make room for the head. They'll be in the same orientation, however.

Stand back and look at the body after making your initial light sketch. What adjustments might you make? Are the legs bigger than the head? Are the arms attached at the shoulders? What's too big? Too small? Out of place? Make your adjustments now.

Now draw the skin. This layer can be the color of the skin or you can leave the skin unpainted for the mother's skin to show through the outline. The second layer can be the outline or the color that "shadows" the outline and merges with bare skin.

Add the umbilical cord from the center of baby's belly. Know where the cord goes, but it may be partially hidden, so plan how it will lie on or behind the limbs.

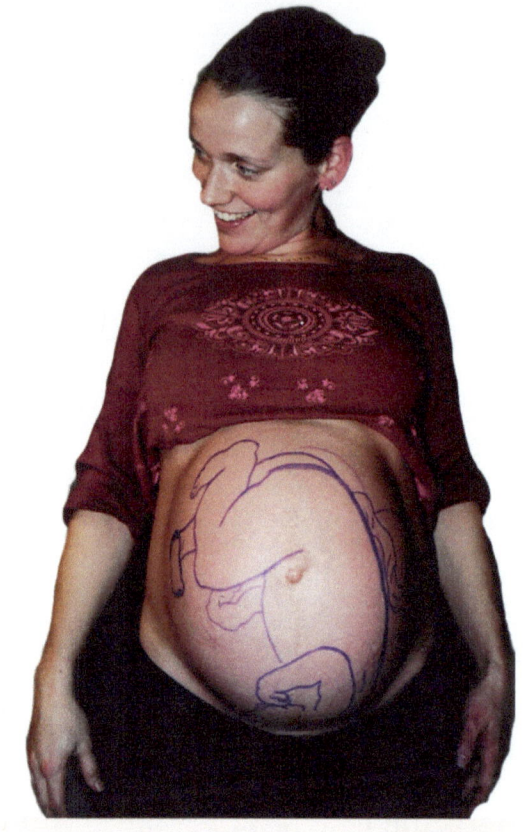

Katie's baby was so easy to feel. The wrist was bent, and I could feel the bend in the elbow. I even heard the umbilical cord!

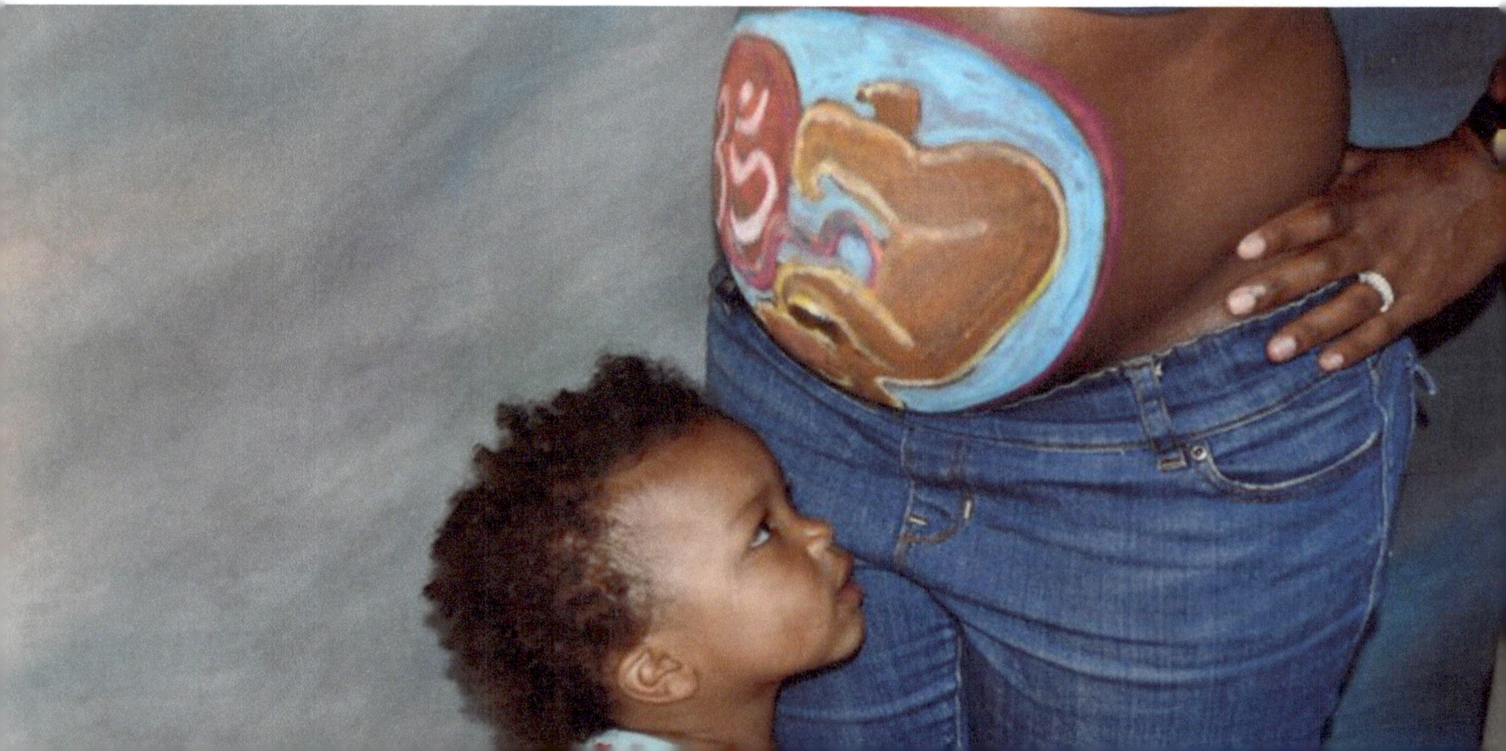

The Limbs

The knees bend toward the belly. Drawing feet tucked into crossed legs is tricky. The elbow(s) will bend similarly to the knees, but smaller, and they're not positioned beyond the knees. Arms and legs are short compared to a child's; a baby can only touch the top of their head with a significant bend at the side.

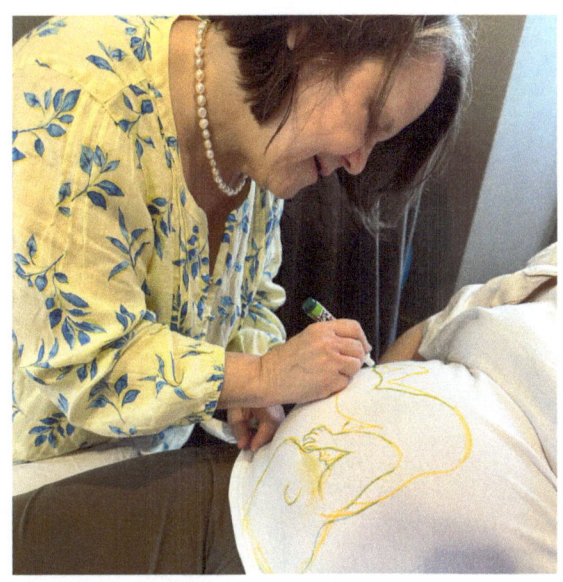

Hands can be near the mouth or ear or on the lap. It can be cute to draw baby with an "A-OK" gesture, a waving hand, or a peace sign. If you feel less than confident about drawing hands, tuck the hands out of sight or soften the details.

Draw the feet smaller than they feel because when they press out, they raise a great deal of womb, fat, and skin over them. The feet are about a third of the length of the leg. The top of the foot can easily touch the shin when the baby fills the womb.

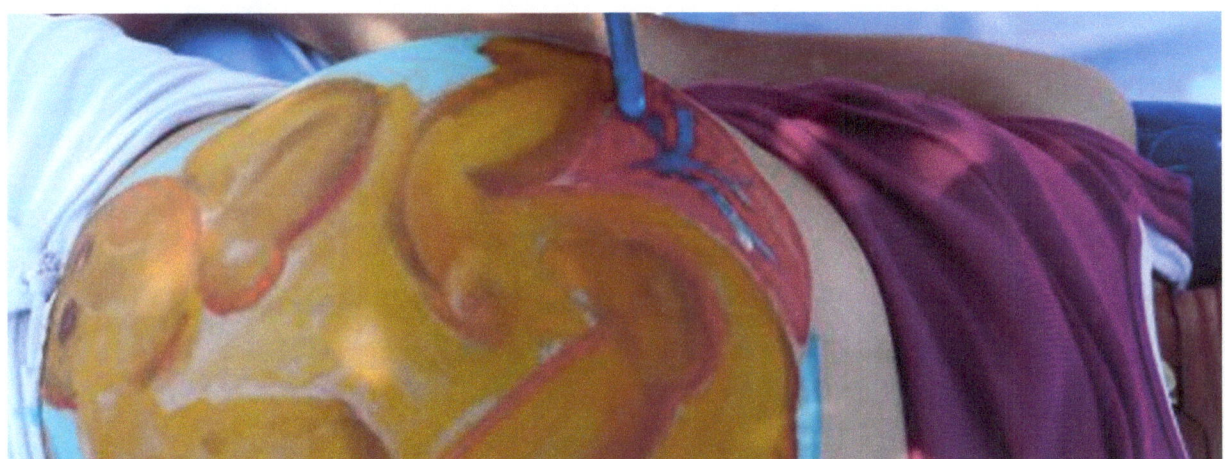

Here's an early attempt at portraying a posterior baby with its limbs in front. I began with the limbs in their actual places. When it came time to draw the head, I realized that most of the head was beneath her pants.

I used to fill in baby's whole body with paint. On the next pages, you will see that I began to incorporate the mother's skin color into baby's skin color.

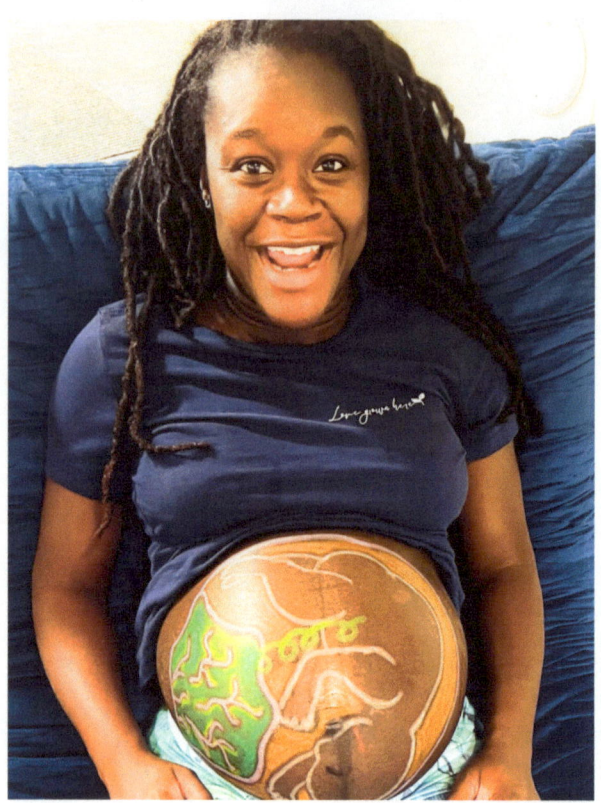

Coloring In the Baby

Now, choose the main color(s) of your baby and go more boldly over the earlier sketch. Use shading for depth, or keep consistent "flat" colors.

If you are painting in all the spaces, paint the broad spaces first. You'll paint the outline after this paint dries. Wait for the paint on the broad bits to dry before you draw in the details. You might dab the very wet areas with a tissue carefully.

I like to use two complementary colors for depth and light. If time or preference only allows one color, pick a contrasting color. Match or complement the color of clothing or skin tones, or ask parents for their color preference.

Jessica Freedman a Spinning Babies® Certified Parent Educator and Daily Essentials Instructor, chose colors of joy for her client.

Add a "Frame" to Represent the Border of the Uterus

Add a border by following the outer edges of the womb with a circle of color. This circle frames the baby. You may choose a realistic or symbolic, anatomical or floral frame. A symbol may occur to you. Let your intuition connect to mother and child, following clues the mother may provide. The frame "cradles" your painting. Paint the background first, but maintain the light tracing created in the previous step. Resist the urge to draw dark or bold.

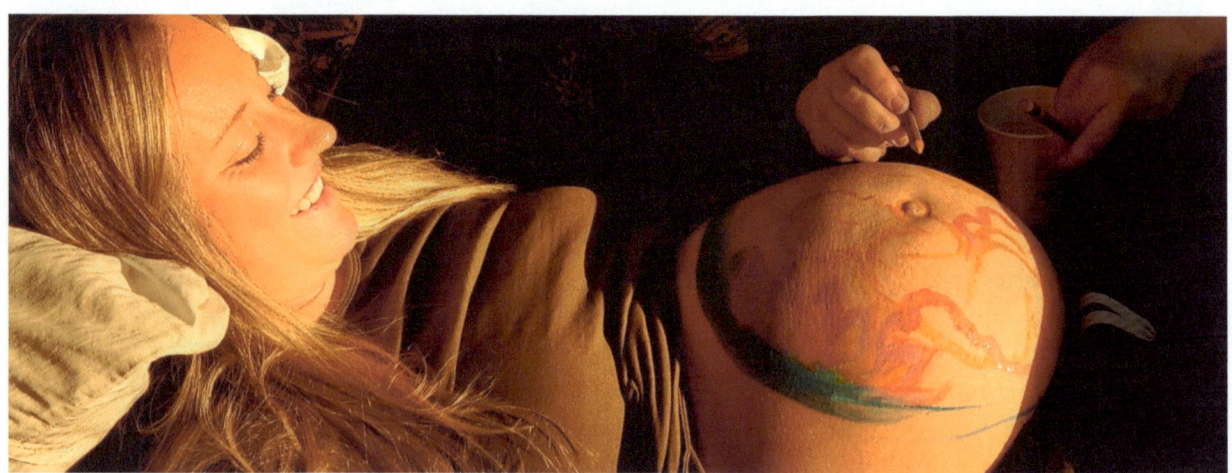

The Placenta

Draw the placenta with more subtle colors than the baby so the baby is emphasized. Often, the placenta is behind the baby. If the placenta is in front of the baby, it's sensible not to include it or draw it behind anyway.

Shape the round edges by using lights and darks. The cord could be bluer than this image.

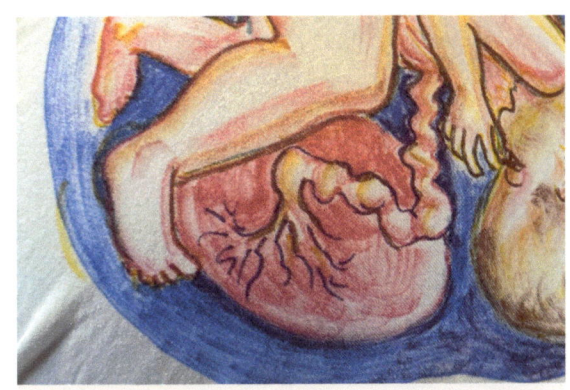

Placentas are a bit of an art form themselves and take practice.

Paint the Protective Amniotic Fluid

The amniotic fluid is a common background. Thin the paint for a light coating. If too wet, you'll have drips. Too dry and you'll pull the abdominal skin.

I wet a blue crayon long enough for it to be soft on the tip.

I had a few drops of water in my brush and simply swirled the brush on the blue crayon to make this transparent and gradient blue amniotic fluid.

Each artist finds their style, and each baby invites individual interpretation.

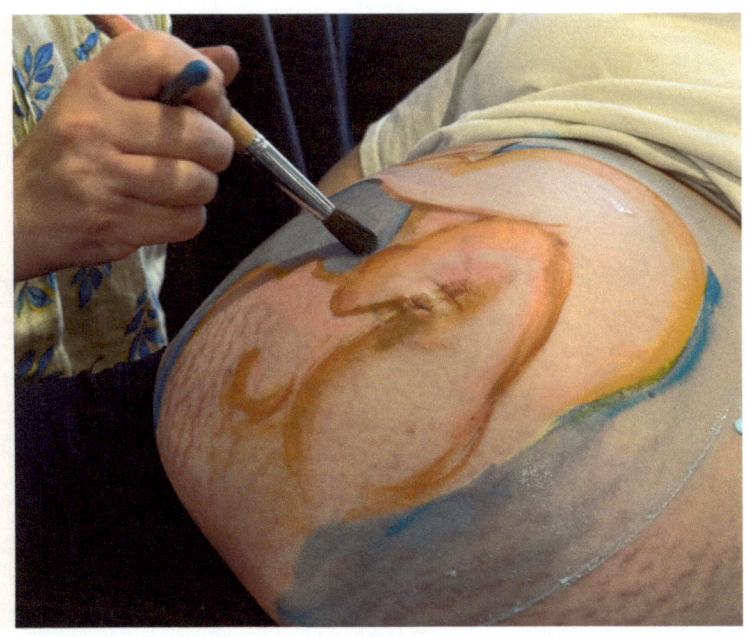

Outlining

Consider an outline after the paint dries to make the illustration show more dramatically. Don't outline over the eyes if they are on the edge of the face. Thicker lines go only on the parts of the baby that are close to the surface. Let the distant parts have thinner lines, or blur the distant portions and sharpen what is close.

You can show close with brighter colors and far with duller.

The Final Details

The final stage is the details of the face, the eyes, and the lips. Eyelashes and the reflected light on the eyes go on after the main part of the face dries.
Highlights are subtle and drawn with a light touch. Anything white (not recommended) is painted last.
Flourishes and details finish the portrait.

Below, glitter is a final touch. Step back and take a look from a distance. You will see what's needed.

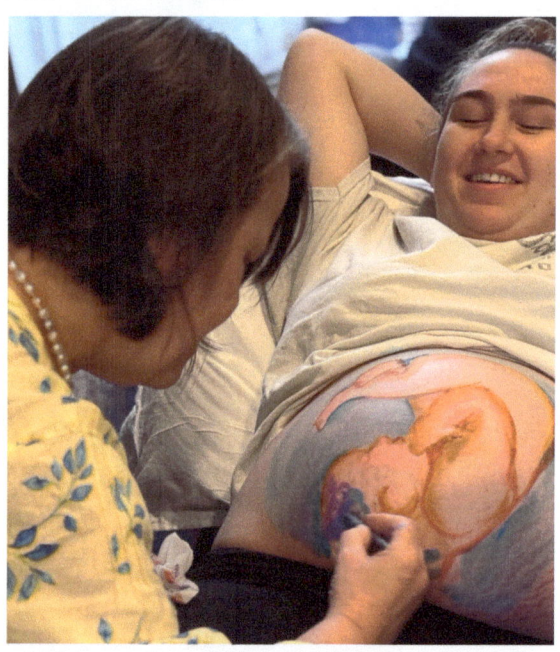

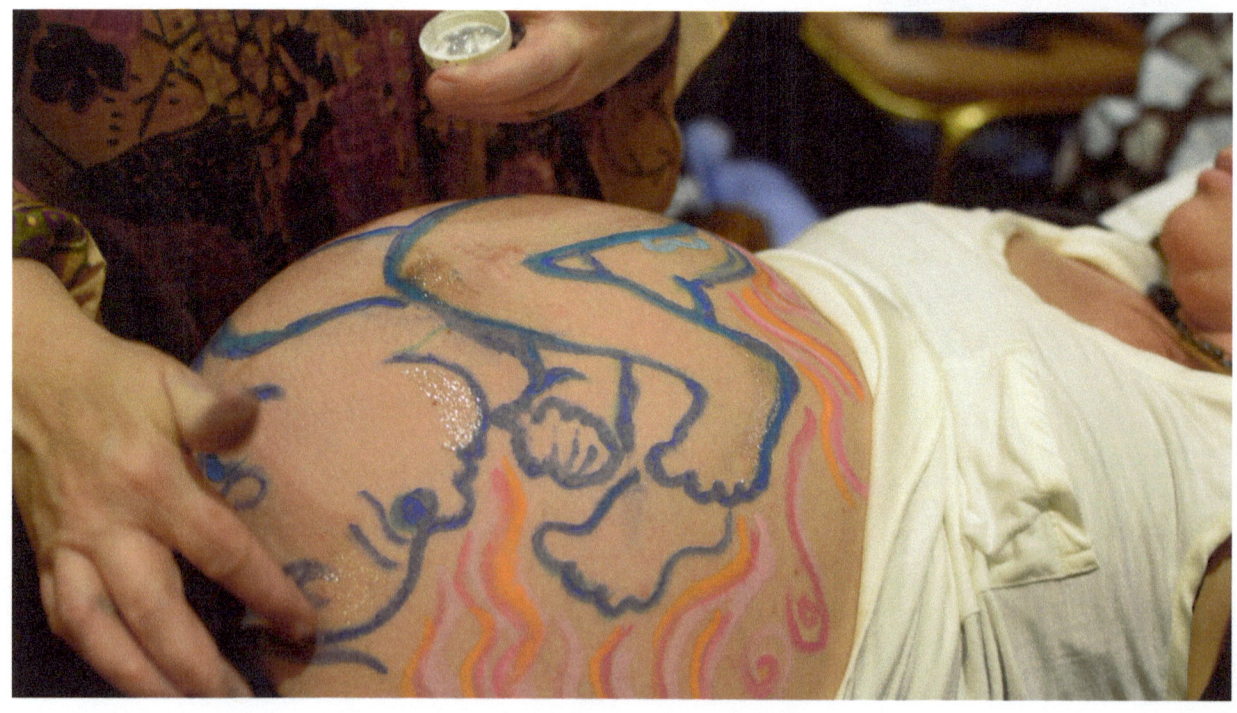

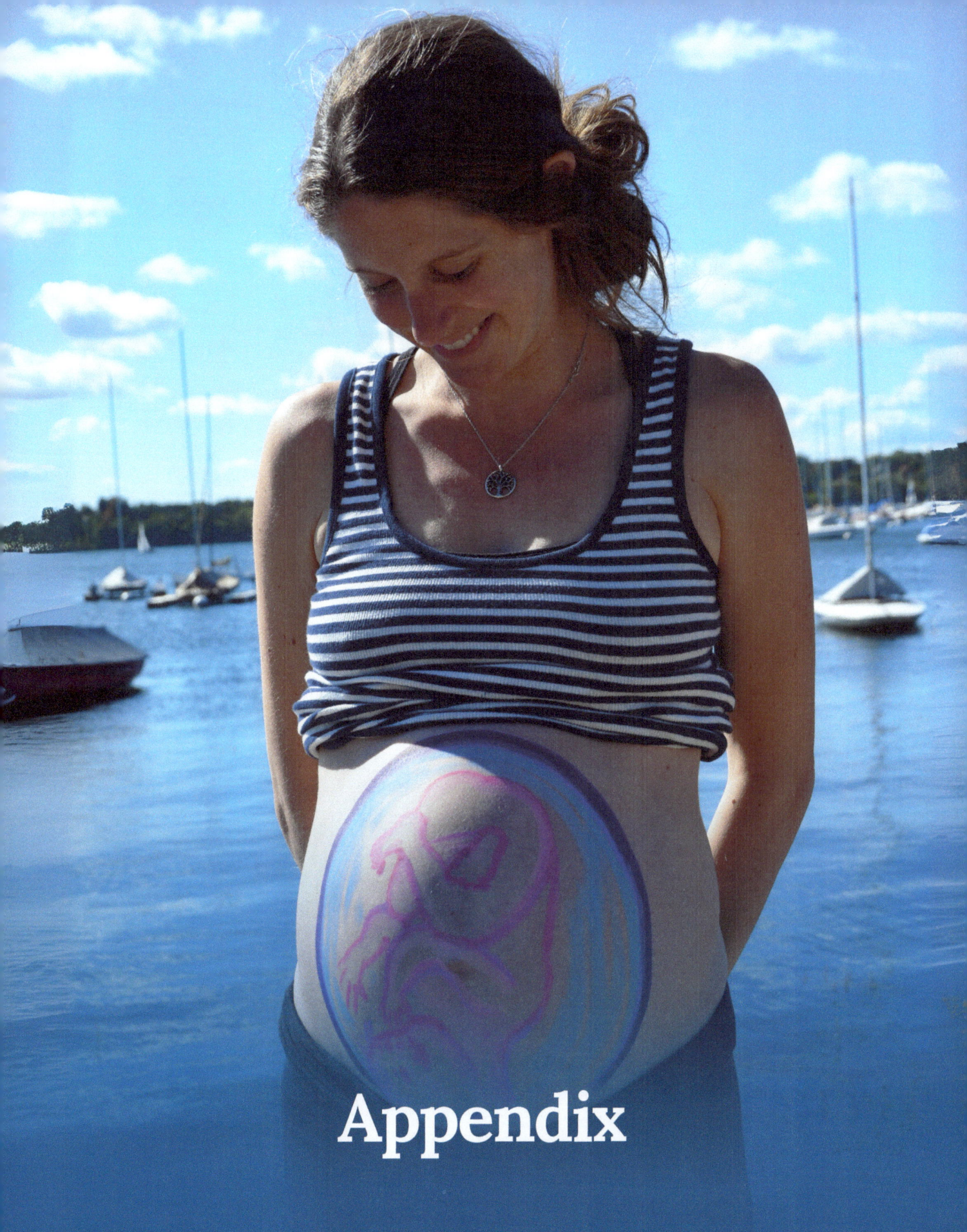

Appendix

The Belly Mapping® Method Template

Your turn!

Position Name
1. _____   2. _____   3. _____   Date ___/___/___

Here is what I feel in my upper right side

Here is what I feel in my upper left side

Your navel may be higher or lower than the center. This depends on the size of your uterus.

Here is what I feel in my lower right side

Here is what I feel in my lower left side

Make lines to show the parts of your baby that you can feel. The left side of your belly appears on the right side of your paper.

Step One: Map the Kicks and Wiggles
(1. Draw a line for the firm, smooth back.
⌒   2. A curve for the bulge at the top.
ᶠ   3. A zigzag or letter K for a kick.
W   4. A W for a wiggle (a softer "kick" area).
♥   5. Place a heart in the area where you or your caregiver hears the baby's heartbeat.
○   6. Make a circle for the baby's head. Your caregiver can help you find the head.

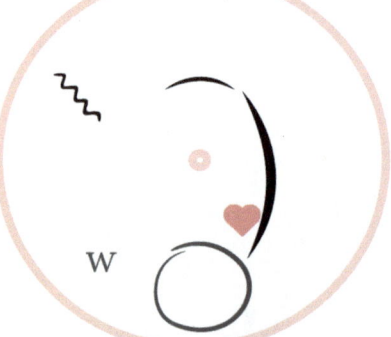

A sample map. The large line on the left marks baby's back (we see it on our right). The kicks are in the upper right. A W shows where the hand wiggles. There is a light gray, curved line for the head that was felt deep in the abdomen with the midwife's help.

Photographing the Painting
Taking a picture or video is the only way to preserve the belly painting. Take a photo with the parent's phone or camera or, if on yours, transfer the pictures to the parent's phone, then either delete them from your camera or obtain written permission from the parents to use the pics on your social media or any other publication.

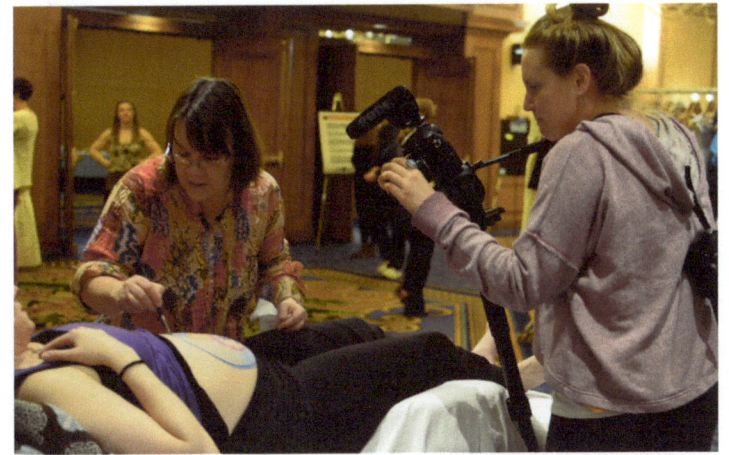

Sharing Your Pictures
Please post the favorite pictures that you have permission to share. Send pics and documentation of permission for use to post on The Belly Mapping® Method page on Facebook. We'd love to feature your pics and stories.

Sharing these pictures of belly painting spreads loving images of pregnancy and the baby within. Tag @SpinningBabies and #BellyMapping to share photos.

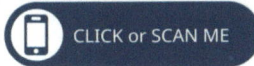

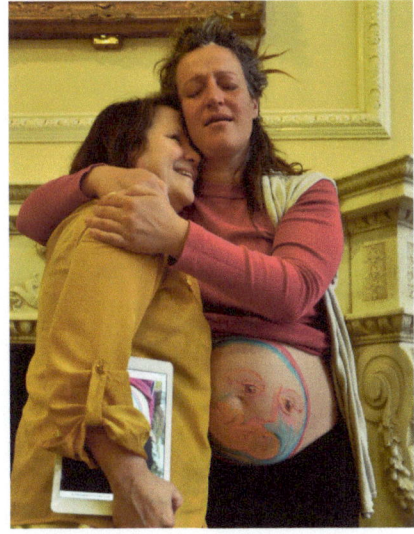

"I was going through a difficult personal time, and I was afraid that my baby was suffering too much from that. So you drew this and made me feel easier and less stressed." —Willma AK

The Belly Mapping® Method as Catharsis
Pregnancy and parenting don't always begin with romance or eagerness.

Sometimes creative, sometimes chaotic, every new child brings change to our relationships, economics, and daily life. Adjustment is seldom instantaneous, but rather a process or a dance.

Social interactions shape our view of ourselves to ourselves. Pregnancy is a sensitive period of social learning for how we care for our child and also for ourselves. How others respond to us helps us form our internal answers to "Who am I now?"

The transformational support from The Belly Mapping® Method is enhanced by our high regard for the mother who is in a period of self-discovery.

Deep connection is the true art of Belly Mapping®.

Spinning Babies® for Easier Birth

Spinning Babies® provides free and for-sale books and classes to help parents and professionals in physiological birth as it relates to baby positions and birth.

"Spinning" simply refers to the turns baby makes to enter and slip through the pelvis during childbirth. When a breech baby turns head down, some say it *spun*!

A baby's position isn't random. Positions and conditions improve as you create space, suppleness, and alignment in your body. Learn how to release tight or twisted muscles and ligaments to experience the easier birth you intend.

There is a "Spectrum of Ease" in birth, and each person begins at a point based on their own history. Falls; car or bike accidents; repeated twists, such as in golf or tennis; or overexercise can mean someone starts on the challenging side of the spectrum. Body balancing throughout pregnancy may help. On the easy side of the spectrum, some people get their desired results when trying balancing activities for the first time in labor.

Birth positions open a portion of the pelvis called a "diameter." Think of these as shaped openings at three levels of the pelvis. Spinning Babies® has changed the way birth positions are chosen. Pelvic Levels Solutions℠ reduce the time that labor takes and reduce the pain from tight muscles or poor positions.

- Meet with a **Spinning Babies® Certified Parent Educator** and take an in-person class with your birth partner and get individual attention.
- Get **bodywork** with a **Spinning Babies® Aware Practitioner**.
- Take our **Birth Prep Online Course** for an overview of Spinning Babies®.
- Stream our **Parent Class video**.
- Pour a cup of pregnancy tea and browse the **Spinning Babies® website**. Begin on the left side of the navigation bar and click through (and if this seems massive, ask your Spinning Babies® Certified Parent Educator for help.
- Find our bonus **Belly Mapping® Method resources here**.

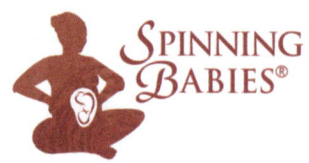

The Belly Mapping® Method Book Resources
Find the templates, links list, and more helpful materials mentioned in this book on our resource page.

Ordering The Belly Mapping® Method Book
Our book is available in both print and e-book.

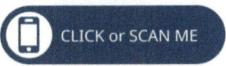

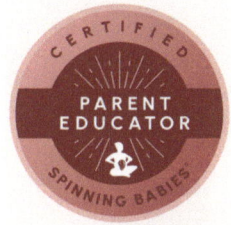
Find a Spinning Babies® Certified Parent Educator
Be guided personally through the Spinning Babies® approach and activities in books, in person, and online.

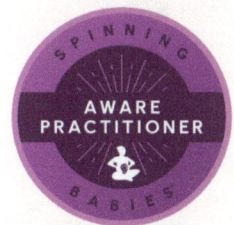
Find a Spinning Babies® Aware Practitioner
Get prenatal bodywork from a Spinning Babies® Aware Practitioner for your baby's position or pregnancy comfort.

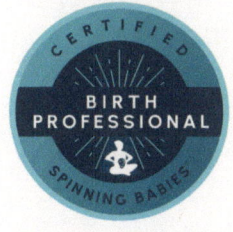
Find a Spinning Babies® Certified Birth Professional
Through the Spinning Babies® lens, these certified birth professionals offer in-the-moment support for comfort and progress in labor.

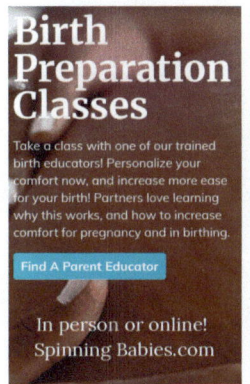
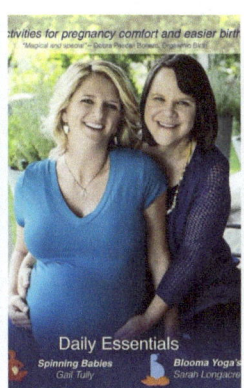
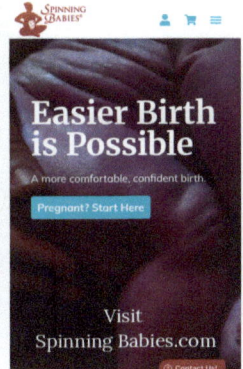
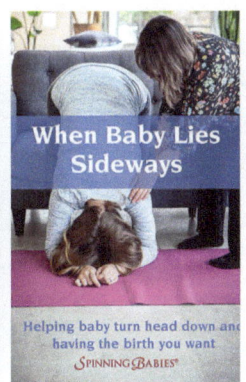
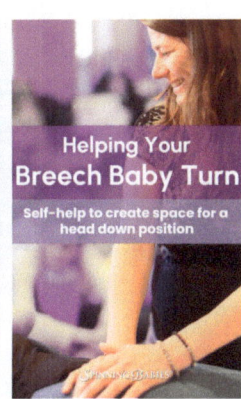

www.spinningbabies.com/shop

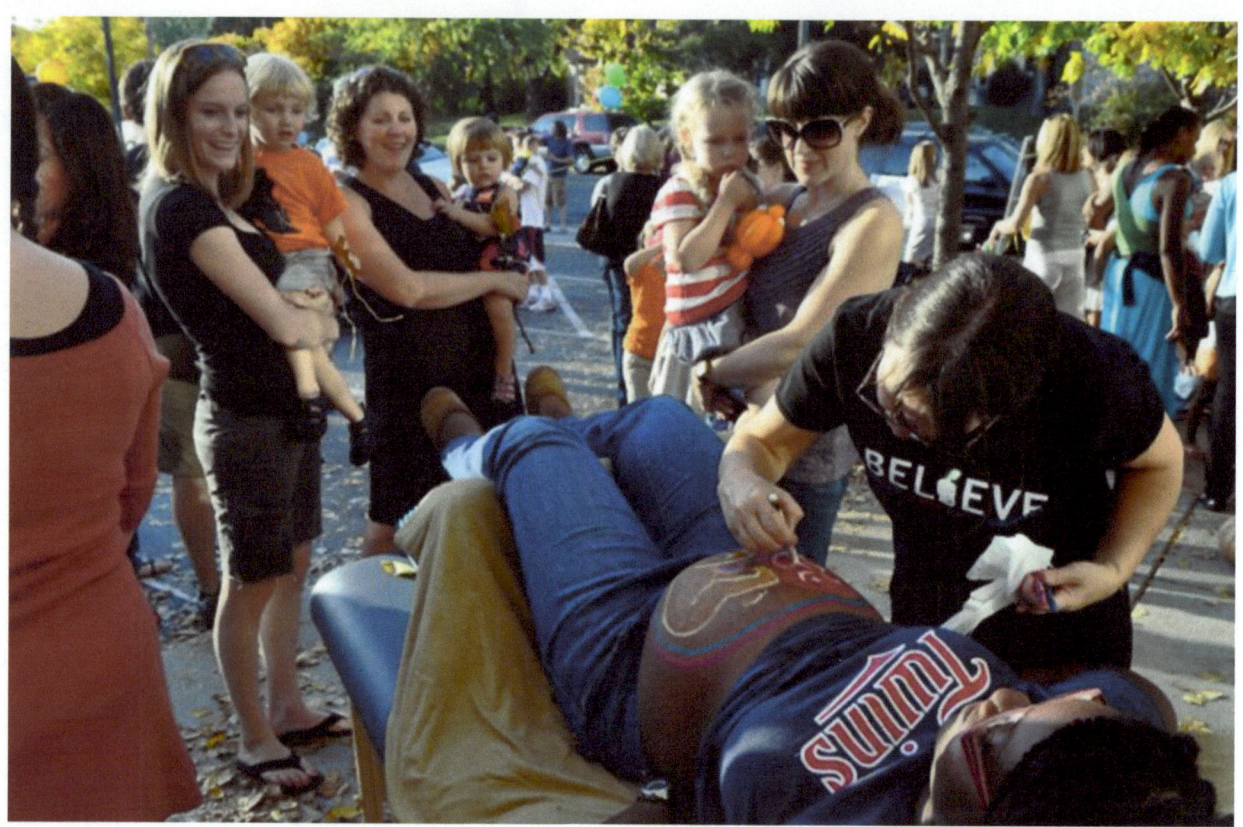

Belly Mapping® in Your Town

Whether you want personal help understanding your baby's position or you want to promote The Belly Mapping® Method at a Baby Fair or other event, we do have someone to help. A Spinning Babies® Certified Parent Educator is trained in The Belly Mapping® Method. They won't feel your belly and make a diagnosis on baby's position; that would be something to ask your care provider. But they can guide you through doing the process yourself.

Can You Do The Belly Mapping® Method with Your Clients?

Yes, individually. But be careful. By saying you do The Belly Mapping® Method, you're not using a verb, you're using a brand name. To use the brand name The Belly Mapping® Method when describing "what you do," you need a license from the owner of the trademark, Spinning Babies®.

Please do this process one-on-one with clients! You cannot, however, use the name, steps, and jingles to promote your business with our company brand. Just like you can pass a Coke to someone, but your company can't serve a drink and call it Coke unless it *is* actually a Coke, and the Coca-Cola Company makes you get a license.

Experience a Personal Guide to The Belly Mapping® Method.
Find someone to work with at SpinningBabies.com/parents/spbcpe-directory.

Glossodex

Glossodex

Abdominal Lift and Tuck A position to engage baby in the top of the pelvis with a contraction. A combination of belly lift and posterior pelvic tilt. 76
acupuncture A therapeutic modality in which needles are inserted into specific parts of the body in order to heal or relieve pain. Used for breech and posterior. 63
amniotic fluid The liquid surrounding the baby in the womb. 15
anterior Toward the front of the body. The anterior position places the baby's occiput (and usually their spine, too) toward the mother's front. 22
body balancing Various bodywork methods, such as chiropractic, craniosacral, and fascial release, that bring about a tensile balance in the fascia. Will enhance function and help the baby into a position to complement the birthing process. 88
bodywork, bodyworkers Physical therapy, massage, or light touch for well-being or balance. 112
breech Baby is positioned buttocks, knees, or feet first. Only about 3–4 percent of babies are breech at the due date of 40 weeks. 8, 54
breech tilt An inversion position resting on one's back, supported by a plank. 62
cardinal movements The series of positions and turns and tucks a baby makes during labor to fit the smallest diameters of the pelvis. 71
care provider, provider, caregiver Professionals who offer primary care for pregnancy and birth, primarily midwives and doctors who are responsible for practice decisions. Does not technically include nurses, doulas. 7
cervical ripening A natural or artificial process to soften and thin the cervix before labor. Collagen fibers dissolve in the cervix. 29
cervix, cervical Latin for neck. The opening of the womb to the vagina. 27
cesarean, cesarean section, c-section A surgical birth from an incision made through the abdomen. The pregnant uterus is cut open and the baby is extracted. 72
craniosacral therapy A holistic practice where a therapist's palpation releases restrictions in the craniosacral system to improve the functioning of the central nervous system. A type of bodywork. Included in many types of fascia therapy. 88
Daily Activities When capitalized, we mean the Spinning Babies® selection of stretches and activities to create suppleness by lengthening muscle fibers and improving range of motion in pregnancy. A page by this name is on our website. 86
doula A Greek word used for a person who supports birthing individuals and couples with childbirth. Dozens of control studies show excellent physical and psychological benefits of doula support. There are also postpartum doulas. 90
engage(d), engagement The baby's head enters the pelvic brim. Also called lightening, or the phrase, the baby "dropped." A cardinal movement. 7
epidural A form of regional anesthesia injected into the space between the epidural membrane and the spine during labor and birth for pain relief. 74
extended, extension Muscles stretched, as when neck muscles extend to lift the chin away from the chest. The back arches and the chest comes forward. 7

Glossodex

exaggerated lateral decumbent When lying on one's side, the person leans forward with their top leg placed upon a pillow or birth ball to make the hips asymmetrical. 76

external cephalic version (ECV) A maneuver where a trained provider attempts to manually turn a breech baby by pressing on the pregnant abdomen. Risks in the procedure make fetal monitoring crucial. Done after baby's lungs are mature in case the placenta detaches, requiring emergency cesarean. 63

fascia Connective tissue uniting the body from under the skin to the bone marrow. Bone, muscles, and organs are made of, connected with, and covered with variations of fascia. Fascia can be fibrous or flexible and comes in sheaths, wraps, ligaments (ropes), hammocks, or bone. Fascia can include nerves, receptors, fluids, and fibrils. Lack of movement creates thicker areas and pain. 63

fascial release A holistic method of releasing the tension in the fascia, the connective membranes surrounding all muscles, organs, bones, and vessels. 88

false labor "Practice" contractions that do not signal the actual beginning of labor; in other words, there is no cervical change, or very little. May be caused by hormones; fetal or maternal activity, such as baby turning; or dehydration. 88

fetal rotation, rotate, rotation The turning movements a baby completes to fit the pelvis and descend during labor and birth. The word spinning in Spinning Babies® highlights fetal rotation. 71

fetoscope A stethoscope to hear the fetus in the womb from 14 or 20 weeks on. 8

finger pads The fleshy surface of the first joint of the fingers (rather than the fingertips). Where your fingerprints are. 13

flexion, flexed Moved toward the center of the body. Bent, curled, as in when the chin is flexed to the chest. The flexed baby's head will fit better. 7

Forward-leaning Inversion Originating with Dr. Carol Phillips, DC, a self-care body balancing technique to allow the uterus to hang from its ligaments. Read up on benefits and risks to avoid harm. One of The Three Balances℠ of Spinning Babies® included with Dr. Carol Phillips's permission. 62

frontum The brow or forehead. Used for a brow presentation. 48

fundus The top of the uterus. Contractions originate in the area of the fundus. 8

head-down baby Any head-down presentation, fetus is positioned head first. 19

homeopathy Holistic treatment based on the concept that "like cures like." 88

Leopold's Maneuvers, Leopold's A four-step hand placement system to determine fetal position by palpation (feeling) through the abdomen. 7

ligament A fibrous strand or filaments of fascia (connective tissue) linking bones through joints and sheaths, connecting organs, or organs to bones. The ovary is connected to the uterus with a suspensory fold of the peritoneum (also fascia). Uterine ligaments uniquely are imbedded with muscle cells so they can grow. 89

linea nigra A line of darkened pigment seen on most pregnant abdomens. 8

maternal positioning Postures and movements to use gravity during pregnancy and labor to guide the baby into an optimal position and open the pelvis. 87

Maya uterine massage An external massage to guide the womb into its optimal position, allowing baby to move into an optimal position. 88

mentum Latin for chin, this is the presenting part of a face presentation. 48

midpelvis The middle channel of the pelvis, at the ischial spines. 71

Glossodex

moxibustion A mugwort coal heating an acupuncture point on the outside, upper corner of the little toe of the pregnant person to turn a breech (or posterior) baby. 88

natural birth Birth without pain medication or other significant medical intervention. Now termed *physiologic birth*. 89

occiput A plate of bone that makes up the back of the skull. The "landmark" for a head-down baby who is not face or forehead first. 48

oblique lie Baby is lying diagonally across the abdomen; the head is by a hip. 15

Open-knee Chest position A birth position used to help rotate a posterior baby or turn a breech in pregnancy. Opens the inlet. The knees are only hip-width apart, not wide "open." Open means the angle of the knees is far from the abdomen. 62

optimal fetal positioning Origin of the term and concept by Jean Sutton and Pauline Scott. Gravity-friendly positions and use of a pregnancy belt to help guide a baby to a flexed presentation (chin is tucked), which includes occiput anterior, left occiput anterior, or left occiput transverse fetal positions with the intent of a straightforward labor experience. 82

palpation To feel the body with one's hands; feeling a baby through the belly. 7

pelvic brim The entrance to the bony pelvis, which a baby must enter to "engage" and begin descent. Walcher's position opens the pelvic brim. 60

pelvic floor A hammock of muscle layers that support abdominal organs. The opening in the pelvic floor allows the urethra, rectum, and vagina through and plays an important role in fetal rotation. Tension or asymmetry in the pelvic floor can lead to malpositioning of the womb and baby. The pelvic floor can be released in pregnancy and labor with a fascial release technique. 63

pelvic outlet The bottom of the pelvis, which a baby must exit before birth. Squatting on flat feet with a posterior pelvic tilt opens the pelvic outlet. 79

perinatal The period from the start of pregnancy through the first year. 4

physiology The interacting functions of biology and anatomy. 82

placenta The "life-support" organ for the baby. Forms in the uterine lining. 7

posterior pelvic tilt Flattening the lower back to bring the top of the pelvis back. The tailbone tucks underneath. A posterior pelvic tilt opens the top of the pelvis. 76

posterior position, posterior Toward the back. The fetal occiput aims toward the back of the pelvis. Also called spine-to-spine, OP, and sunny-side up. 29

presenting, presentation The part of the baby coming through the pelvis first is presenting. The position of the baby with an added detail of flexion or extension. 7

psoas ("sō-ăz") A nerve-laced muscle pair allowing us to stand upright. Originating from the spine under the diaphragm, coming over the front pelvis to attach to the top of the leg. 78

pubic bone, symphysis pubis The joint and cartilage joining the arch between the hip bones—the pubic arch. In the front of the pelvis, beneath the pubic hair. 8

Glossodex

right obliquity A common orientation of the uterus making the right side higher and steeper. 74

round ligaments Ligaments that anchor and support the womb in the front. They attach to the fascia on the pubic arch, which is the lower border of the pubic bone to the start of the sitz bones. 63

sacrum, sacral The triangular bone at the base of the spine. The "slide" for baby during pushing. The tailbone connects to the sacrum and can open like a door as the head passes by; relating to the sacrum, as in craniosacral, a method of bodywork. 48

Side-ying Release Originating with Dr. Carol Phillips, DC, a body balancing technique with benefits for pelvic floor comfort, range of motion, and fetal rotation. One of The Three Balances^{SM}. 77

spectrum of ease A concept to bring people away from either/or thinking of one best technique. 70

spontaneous birth, spontaneous onset of labor Birth allowed to begin and continue naturally, without induction or augmentation from external substances, and end without forceps, vacuum, ventouse, or cesarean. 89

starting position Baby's position just prior to labor, or in latent labor. 73

third trimester The last third of pregnancy from 28 weeks to birth. 15

transition Active labor is often divided into two parts, active labor and transition phase, and both are part of the first stage of labor. Often 7–10 cm dilation, characterized by long, strong contractions.

transverse lie The position in which a baby lies horizontally across a womb. In labor, this baby could then have a shoulder presentation or an arm could come out first. If the baby can't be helped to head down or breech, the birth will have to be by cesarean. 15

ultrasound, sonogram Ultrasonic waves to acquire an image inside the body. In childbearing, to image the fetus, or to listen to the fetal heart rate by an electronic external fetal monitor. 8

uterine ligaments The ligaments supporting and connecting the womb. See round ligaments. 87

uterine torsion A twist in the lower uterus from a sudden stop while turning, such as in sports, that reduces the space available and disrupts the regularity and aim of the uterine contractions. 16

vertical lie The spine of the fetus is in the same direction of the pregnant person's spine. 15

Webster Maneuver (technique) Dr. Webster, DC, popularized a sequence of techniques that increase the spontaneous flipping of the breech fetus to cephalic, or head down. It involves a sacroiliac joint adjustment along with a round ligament release on the opposite side. 63